Urology

Editors

GRETCHEN M. IRWIN
LAURA MAYANS

PRIMARY CARE: CLINICS IN OFFICE PRACTICE

www.primarycare.theclinics.com

Consulting Editor
JOEL J. HEIDELBAUGH

June 2019 • Volume 46 • Number 2

ELSEVIER

1600 John F. Kennedy Boulevard • Suite 1800 • Philadelphia, Pennsylvania, 19103-2899

http://www.theclinics.com

PRIMARY CARE: CLINICS IN OFFICE PRACTICE Volume 46, Number 2
June 2019 ISSN 0095-4543, ISBN-13: 978-0-323-67807-0

Editor: Jessica McCool
Developmental Editor: Laura Fisher

Primary Care: Clinics in Office Practice (ISSN: 0095-4543) is published quarterly by Elsevier Inc., 360 Park Avenue South, New York, NY 10010-1710. Months of issue are March, June, September, and December. Periodicals postage paid at New York, NY and additional mailing offices. Subscription prices are $246.00 per year (US individuals), $505.00 (US institutions), $100.00 (US students), $303.00 (Canadian individuals), $572.00 (Canadian institutions), $175.00 (Canadian students), $357.00 (international individuals), $572.00 (international institutions), and $175.00 (international students). Foreign air speed delivery is included in all *Clinics* subscription prices. All prices are subject to change without notice. POSTMASTER: Send address changes to *Primary Care: Clinics in Office Practice*, Elsevier Periodicals Customer Service, 11830 Westline Industrial Drive, St. Louis, MO 63146. Customer Service Health Sciences Division, Subscription Customer Service, 3251 Riverport Lane, Maryland Heights, MO 63043. **Customer Service: 1-800-654-2452 (U.S. and Canada); 314-447-8871 (outside U.S. and Canada). Fax: 314-447-8029. E-mail: journalscustomerservice-usa@elsevier.com (for print support); journalsonlinesupport-usa@elsevier.com (for online support).**

Reprints. For copies of 100 or more, of articles in this publication, please contact the Commercial Reprints Department, Elsevier Inc., 360 Park Avenue South, New York, NY 10010-1710. Tel. 212-633-3874; Fax: 212-633-3820; E-mail: reprints@elsevier.com.

Primary Care: Clinics in Office Practice is covered in *MEDLINE/PubMed (Index Medicus) and EMBASE/Excerpta Medica, Current Contents/Clinical Medicine, and ISI/BIOMED.*

Contributors

CONSULTING EDITOR

JOEL J. HEIDELBAUGH, MD, FAAFP, FACG
Clinical Professor, Departments of Family Medicine and Urology, University of Michigan Medical School, Ann Arbor, Michigan

EDITORS

GRETCHEN M. IRWIN, MD, MBA, FAAFP
Associate Professor with Tenure, Department of Family and Community Medicine, KU School of Medicine-Wichita, Wichita, Kansas

LAURA MAYANS, MD, MPH
Clinical Assistant Professor, Department of Family and Community Medicine, KU School of Medicine-Wichita, Wichita, Kansas

AUTHORS

FERESHTEH GERAYLI, MD
Professor of Family Medicine, Faculty member, Johnson City Family Medicine Residency Program, East Tennessee State University Quillen College of Medicine, ETSU Family Medicine Associates, Johnson City, Tennessee

MARIS HOKE, MD
Assistant Professor, Department of Community and Family Medicine, University of Missouri-Kansas City, Kansas City, Missouri

JAMES D. HOLT, MD
Professor of Family Medicine, Associate Program Director, Johnson City Family Medicine Residency Program, East Tennessee State University Quillen College of Medicine, ETSU Family Medicine Associates, Johnson City, Tennessee

MIRANDA M. HUFFMAN, MD, MEd
Associate Professor, Department of Family and Community Medicine, Meharry Medical College, Nashville, Tennessee

GRETCHEN M. IRWIN, MD, MBA, FAAFP
Associate Professor with Tenure, Department of Family and Community Medicine, KU School of Medicine-Wichita, Wichita, Kansas

KARYN B. KOLMAN, MD
Vice Chair Education, Assistant Professor, Department of Family and Community Medicine, University of Arizona College of Medicine–Tucson, Tucson, Arizona

ROBERT C. LANGAN, MD, FAAFP
Program Director, St. Luke's Family Medicine Residency, Sacred Heart Campus, Allentown, Pennsylvania; Adjunct Associate Professor, Department of Family and Community Medicine, Temple University School of Medicine, Philadelphia, Pennsylvania

LAURA MAYANS, MD, MPH
Clinical Assistant Professor, Department of Family and Community Medicine, KU School of Medicine-Wichita, Wichita, Kansas

LEAH M. PETERSON, MD
Faculty Physician, Smoky Hill Family Medicine Residency Program, Salina, Kansas

HENRY S. REED, MD
Internal Medicine/Nephrology, Mowery Clinic, Salina, Kansas

ANIESA SLACK, MD
Assistant Professor, Department of Community and Family Medicine, University of Missouri-Kansas City, Kansas City, Missouri

JENNIFER E. THUENER, MD
Assistant Professor, Faculty, Department of Family and Community Medicine, The University of Kansas Medical Center, Wichita, Kansas

ROBIN A. WALKER, MD
Department of Family and Community Medicine, Assistant Clinical Professor, KU School of Medicine-Wichita, Wichita, Kansas

Contents

Foreword: To Own the Truth, Own the Data ix

Joel J. Heidelbaugh

Preface: Urologic Commonalities and Challenges xi

Gretchen M. Irwin and Laura Mayans

Cystitis and Pyelonephritis: Diagnosis, Treatment, and Prevention 191

Karyn B. Kolman

Urinary tract infections, including cystitis and pyelonephritis, are the most common bacterial infection primary care clinicians encounter in office practice. Dysuria and frequency in the absence of vaginal discharge and vaginal irritation are highly predictive of cystitis. Urine culture is recommended for the diagnosis and management of pyelonephritis, recurrent urinary tract infection, and complicated urinary tract infections. Antibiotics targeted toward Escherichia coli, Proteus, Klebsiella, and Staphylococcus saprophyticus are the recommended treatment. The duration of treatment varies by specific drug and type of infection, ranging from 3 to 5 days for uncomplicated cystitis to 7 to 14 days for pyelonephritis.

Nephrolithiasis 203

Laura Mayans

Incidence of nephrolithiasis has increased dramatically over the past 30 years, likely due to environmental changes such as dietary habits. Nephrolithiasis presents as acute flank or abdominal pain with nausea and vomiting. Hematuria is present in 90% of cases, but its absence does not rule out nephrolithiasis. Most cases can be managed expectantly as an outpatient with hydration, analgesia, and possibly medications to aide in passage. A metabolic evaluation may be indicated after a second episode of nephrolithiasis in adults or after a first episode in children or those with a family history of nephrolithiasis.

Bladder Pain Syndrome 213

Miranda M. Huffman, Aniesa Slack, and Maris Hoke

Bladder pain syndrome (BPS) is a common cause of chronic pelvic pain with associated lower urinary symptoms. BPS is incurable; management requires an interdisciplinary team (nutritionist, physical therapist, behavioral health specialist) focusing on maximizing patient function. For patients, dietary changes (avoiding acidic, spicy, and caffeinated foods) are effective at relieving symptoms. Medications may be considered in patients who do not respond to these treatments. Referral to urology or urogynecology should be considered if bladder cancer is suspected (especially in patients who smoke or have environmental exposures) and in patients with refractive symptoms for consideration of intravesicular therapy.

Prostate Cancer Screening 257

James D. Holt and Fereshteh Gerayli

Whether to screen for prostate cancer in aging men is a topic that is fairly well researched, but recommendations are controversial, because the evidence supporting any recommendation is equivocal. The evidence clearly does not support routine screening of all average-risk men, but for men aged 55 to 69 years, either not routinely screening, or engaging each man in shared decision making for his individual preference on screening, is reasonable and consistent with the evidence. Many organizations, including the American Cancer Society, have not yet reassessed their guidelines, in response to the US Preventative Services Task Force revised guideline.

Hematuria 265

Leah M. Peterson and Henry S. Reed

Hematuria is common in the primary care setting. It is classified as either gross or microscopic. Hematuria warrants a thorough history and physical to determine potential causes and assess risk factors for malignancy. Risk of malignancy with gross hematuria is greater than 10%, and prompt urologic referral is recommended. Microscopic hematuria most commonly has benign causes, such as urinary tract infection, benign prostatic hyperplasia, and urinary calculi. If no benign cause for microscopic hematuria is found, the work-up includes laboratory tests to rule out intrinsic renal disease, imaging of the urinary tract, and referral to nephrology and urology subspecialists.

Urologic Malignancies 275

Jennifer E. Thuener

The primary care physician should be familiar with renal and bladder cancer risk factors, symptoms, and workup. Bladder cancer generally presents with painless hematuria, which primary care providers may identify. Bladder cancer is treated more successfully when caught early. Patients need support and follow-up through treatment. Renal cell carcinoma is generally asymptomatic and commonly is an incidental finding on abdominal imaging. The workup of incidental renal masses is important and ensure appropriate follow-up and treatment are received. Renal cancer is easier to successfully treat when identified at an early stage, so proper identification is important for appropriate treatment.

PRIMARY CARE: CLINICS IN OFFICE PRACTICE

FORTHCOMING ISSUES

September 2019
Palliative Care
Alan R. Roth, Serife Eti and Peter A. Selwyn, *Editors*

December 2019
Population Health
Devdutta Sangvai and Anthony J. Viera, *Editors*

March 2020
Sports Medicine
Peter J. Carek, *Editor*

RECENT ISSUES

March 2019
Prevention and Screening
Joanna L. Drowos, *Editor*

December 2018
Women's Health
Diane M. Harper and Emily M. Godfrey, *Editors*

September 2018
Infectious Disease
Michael A. Malone, *Editor*

SERIES OF RELATED INTEREST

Urologic Clinics (https://www.urologic.theclinics.com/)
Medical Clinics (http://www.medical.theclinics.com)
Physician Assistant Clinics (http://www.physicianassistant.theclinics.com)

Foreword
To Own the Truth, Own the Data

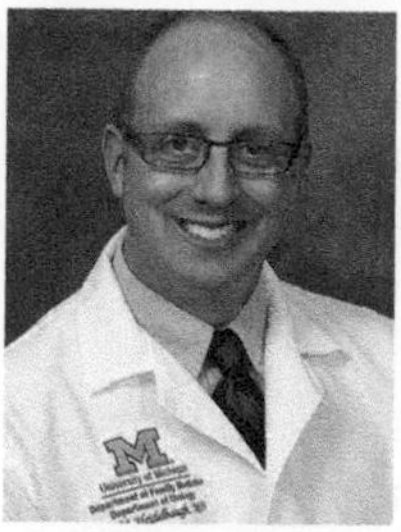

Joel J. Heidelbaugh, MD, FAAFP, FACG
Consulting Editor

Urologic conditions continue to challenge primary care providers with regard to accurate diagnosis and treatment. A middle-aged woman who suffers from "chronic urinary tract infections" and "pyelonephritis" was recently referred to my clinic for evaluation. She stated that she was "tired of always being prescribed antibiotics," many of which she had an adverse reaction to. She admitted that she had been to many doctors and urgent care practices over the last few years in search of answers for her symptoms and was recently told that she must have "stones or some kind of blockage" as the cause of her chronic infections. She had been treated with antibiotics via clinic phone triage, after urgent care encounters, and at many office visits. She almost always had urinalyses performed, most of which were negative to equivocal, and rarely had a urine culture performed, yet never had a positive culture. The concept that she could have anything other than "chronic urinary tract infections" somehow seemed foreign to her, yet an appropriate workup and education offered significant insight into the possibility of a functional rather than an organic disorder.

The advent of phosphodiesterase type 5 inhibitors in the late 1990s revolutionized the treatment of erectile dysfunction for men worldwide. Subsequently, the relationship between erectile dysfunction and endothelial dysfunction has alerted clinicians to the increased risk of underlying cardiovascular disease in men with erectile dysfunction, necessitating a thorough cardiac and metabolic workup in affected men.

Prostate cancer screening remains perhaps one of the most controversial topics in all of medicine. Over 30,000 men die annually from this poorly understood disease, yet many populations of men remain overscreened, overbiopsied, and overtreated without clear models to predict morbidity or mortality. Between 2012 and 2017, when the US Preventive Services Task Force recommended against prostate cancer screening, many cancers went undetected, increasing the risk of metastatic disease. As guidelines change frequently, clinicians remain challenged to provide unbiased shared decision-making practices while educating men.

Prim Care Clin Office Pract 46 (2019) ix–x
https://doi.org/10.1016/j.pop.2019.03.002

Novel advances in treatment for chronic bladder pain syndrome, urinary incontinence, and benign prostatic hyperplasia will provide many patients with options to improve their symptoms and their lives. This issue of *Primary Care: Clinics in Office Practice* highlights these and other common urologic conditions, including enuresis, nephrolithiasis, hematuria, and urologic malignancies.

I would like to thank Drs Mayans and Irwin and their authors on a stellar accomplishment of creating a very practical compendium of articles on common urologic topics that are frequently encountered in primary care practices. Moreover, these articles provide readers with very practical approaches to urologic conditions and how to best educate and guide clinicians and patients toward appropriate shared decision making with regard to screening and testing. To own the truth in diagnostic evaluations, we must own the correct data.

Joel J. Heidelbaugh, MD, FAAFP, FACG
Departments of Family Medicine and Urology
University of Michigan Medical School
Ann Arbor, MI 48103, USA

Ypsilanti Health Center
200 Arnet, Suite 200
Ypsilanti, MI 48198, USA

E-mail address:
jheidel@umich.edu

Preface
Urologic Commonalities and Challenges

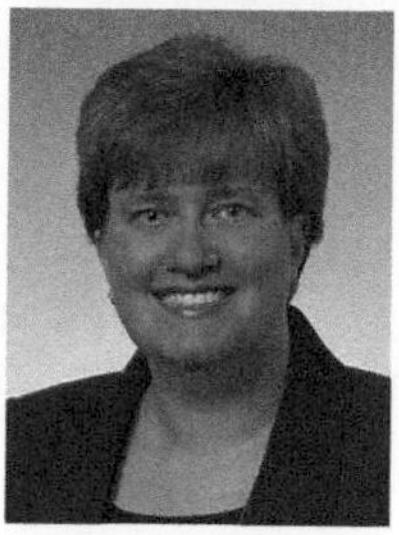

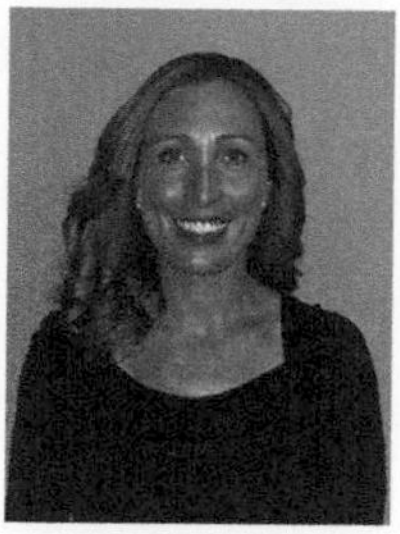

Gretchen M. Irwin, MD, MBA, FAAFP   Laura Mayans, MD, MPH
Editors

From enuresis to incontinence, urologic symptoms can impact individuals of all genders throughout the lifespan. Urologic conditions may cause physical pain or psychological discomfort that can have tremendous negative impact on an individual's well-being. Urologic symptoms, such as dysuria, hematuria, erectile dysfunction, and bladder pain, are common and yet are all too often underreported to primary care physicians. Some patients are embarrassed to discuss symptoms, while others may mistakenly believe that there is no treatment available that can be helpful. Though urologic symptoms are common, treating urologic symptoms may prove to be a challenge for primary care physicians. In some cases, treatment modalities are limited and may not be readily available to all patients. For other conditions, there is no one-size-fits-all solution that can be offered to patients, and the trial and error necessary to find the right treatment may prove frustrating over time. Yet prompt recognition and treatment of urologic concerns may be the key to preventing serious complications and addressing life-threatening conditions while still in the most early and treatable stages. This issue seeks to provide reference for the diagnosis and treatment of common and

Prim Care Clin Office Pract 46 (2019) xi–xii
https://doi.org/10.1016/j.pop.2019.03.001
0095-4543/19/© 2019 Published by Elsevier Inc.

challenging urologic conditions with the goal of improving patient quality of life and overall health.

Gretchen M. Irwin, MD, MBA, FAAFP
University of Kansas School of Medicine - Wichita
1010 North Kansas
Wichita, KS 67214, USA

Laura Mayans, MD, MPH
University of Kansas School of Medicine - Wichita
1010 North Kansas
Wichita, KS 67214, USA

E-mail addresses:
Girwin2@kumc.edu (G.M. Irwin)
lauracmayans@gmail.com (L. Mayans)

Cystitis and Pyelonephritis

Diagnosis, Treatment, and Prevention

Karyn B. Kolman, MD

KEYWORDS

• Urinary tract infection • Recurrent UTI • Pyelonephritis • Cystitis • Prevention • Treatment

KEY POINTS

- Uncomplicated urinary tract infections occur in otherwise healthy, nonpregnant women with normal genitourinary tracts and no recent history of instrumentation, including bladder catheterization.
- The combination of dysuria and frequency in the absence of vaginal discharge and vaginal irritation is more than 90% predictive for cystitis. Symptoms are less reliable in postmenopausal women owing to the high prevalence of chronic urinary complaints.
- Routine use of imaging is not necessary for the diagnosis of uncomplicated cystitis or pyelonephritis.
- The initial antibiotic choice should be based on individual patient factors and local antibiotic resistance patterns. Duration of treatment ranges from 3 to 5 days for uncomplicated cystitis to 7 to 14 days for pyelonephritis.
- There is a need for additional data to support the use of nonantimicrobial prophylaxis for recurrent urinary tract infections.

INTRODUCTION

Urinary tract infections (UTIs) are the most common bacterial infection primary care clinicians will encounter in office practice, accounting for approximately 5 million primary care office visits in 2007.[1] UTIs are much more common in women than in men. During their lifetime, 40% to 50% of women are diagnosed and treated for a UTI, with most being diagnosed before the age of 25.[2]

As health care costs continue to rise and antimicrobial resistance becomes more widespread, clinicians must constantly review and adjust their practice patterns to provide the best, most effective care to their patients and the population as a whole. This review focuses on the diagnosis, treatment, and prevention of the most common UTIs, namely, cystitis and pyelonephritis.

Disclosure Statement: The author has nothing to disclose.

Department of Family and Community Medicine, University of Arizona, College of Medicine – Tucson, 755 N Alvernon Way, Suite 228-230, Tucson, AZ 85711, USA
E-mail address: Karyn.kolman@bannerhealth.com

Prim Care Clin Office Pract 46 (2019) 191–202
https://doi.org/10.1016/j.pop.2019.01.001

DEFINITIONS

UTI is a general term used to designate any infection of the urinary tract and includes asymptomatic bacteriuria, cystitis, and pyelonephritis. Asymptomatic bacteriuria by definition occurs in patients without urinary symptoms who have growth of 10^5 bacteria or more in 2 consecutive urine specimens in women or a single sample in men.[3,4]

Cystitis and pyelonephritis are symptomatic UTIs involving the bladder and kidneys, respectively, and are further classified as uncomplicated or complicated based on risk factors in the affected patient[5] (**Fig. 1**). This classification is aimed to help identify those patients who may need additional diagnostic tests, broader spectrum antibiotics, and/or longer durations of treatment.

An uncomplicated UTI is one that occurs in an otherwise healthy, nonpregnant woman with a normal genitourinary tract and no recent history of instrumentation, including bladder catheterization.[4,6] All other UTIs are classified as complicated. Note that, in this classification system, women with diabetes are automatically classified as having complicated infections. However, many experts would consider women with well-controlled diabetes who otherwise meet the criteria for an uncomplicated infection to have an uncomplicated UTI.[6]

Both cystitis and pyelonephritis may occur as uncomplicated and complicated infections, depending on patient risk factors. Although cystitis can progress to acute pyelonephritis, this occurrence is rare.[7] More commonly, acute pyelonephritis is thought to develop as a primary infection with both patient and bacterial factors playing a role in its occurrence.[8] Complications associated with pyelonephritis include sepsis, acute kidney injury, development of renal or perinephric abscess, and emphysematous pyelonephritis.[9]

Recurrent UTIs are commonly defined as 3 or more infections within a 12-month period or 2 or more infections within a 6-month period.[4,10,11] Of women who have a UTI, 20% to 30% will have a recurrence within 3 months.[10,12]

RISK FACTORS

Premenopausal Women

In young, healthy, premenopausal women, the most common identifiable risk factors for UTI are recent sexual intercourse, spermicide use, and a previous history of UTI.[13]

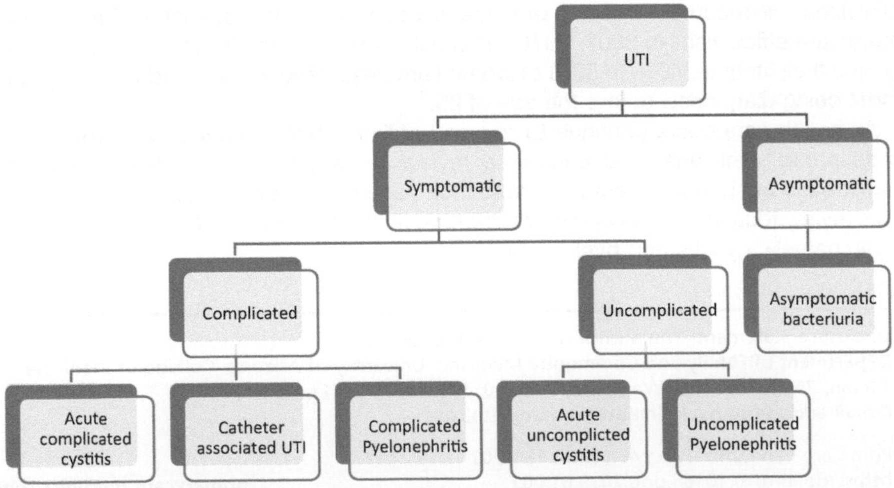

Fig. 1. Classification of UTIs.

Table 1
Summary of risk factors and diagnosis for common UTIs

Type of Infection	Risk Factors	Urine Culture Needed for Diagnosis?
Uncomplicated cystitis		
Premenopausal women	Recent sexual intercourse Spermicide use Previous history of UTI	No
Postmenopausal women	History of UTI Urinary incontinence Cystocele Vaginal prolapse Incomplete bladder emptying	Should be considered if ≤1 symptom present
Pyelonephritis	Recent sexual intercourse Spermicide use Previous history of UTI Mother with UTIs Incontinence women >30 years Diabetes	Yes
Recurrent UTI	Recent sexual intercourse Spermicide use Previous history of UTI Mother with UTIs	Yes, at least once while symptoms are present

Data from Refs.[12–21]

These risk factors also have been identified in women with recurrent cystitis and pyelonephritis.[12] Another significant risk factor for recurrent cystitis and pyelonephritis include a mother with history of UTIs.[14,15] Additionally, pyelonephritis is associated with incontinence in women less than 30 years of age and individuals with diabetes[15] (**Table 1**).

There is no consistent evidence to show that behaviors such as postcoital voiding, hydration status, wiping patterns, tampon use, douching, type of underwear, or use of hot tubs are significantly associated with a risk for recurrent UTIs.[4,14]

Postmenopausal Women

Postmenopausal women are at increased risk of UTI for a number of reasons, including the lower levels of vaginal and systemic estrogen, which is thought to play a role in continence, vaginal pH, and maintaining the normal vaginal flora.[16] Other risk factors for recurrent UTI in postmenopausal women include a history of UTI before menopause, urinary incontinence, cystocele, vaginal prolapse, incomplete bladder emptying, and a change in the vaginal flora.[16,17]

PRESENTATION AND DIAGNOSIS

The clinical presentation of acute cystitis can include dysuria, frequency, urgency, suprapubic pain, and hematuria.[18] Women presenting with a constellation of symptoms consistent with cystitis are more likely to have a culture-proven infection than women presenting with just 1 symptom.[18,19]

The presence of fever, chills, flank pain, nausea, vomiting, and/or costovertebral angle tenderness suggest a diagnosis of pyelonephritis.[15] Pyelonephritis may occur in patients with or without typical urinary symptoms.[4]

Urine culture is the gold standard diagnostic test for all UTIs. However, it may be unnecessary for diagnosis in many situations. The diagnostic workup depends on the type of infection, patient factors, and whether the infection is complicated (see **Table 1**).

Uncomplicated Cystitis

Premenopausal women

Symptomatology alone has a high predictive value of acute cystitis in premenopausal women. Among women who have had at least 1 UTI, self-diagnosis of symptoms correlates with culture-proven UTI greater than 80% of the time.[18] The combination of dysuria and frequency in the absence of vaginal discharge and vaginal irritation has a predictive value for cystitis of more than 90%.[18] In these situations, it is recommended that the diagnosis be made without any confirmatory laboratory testing.[4,20] Urine dipstick testing should be performed when only 1 symptom is present or if nonspecific symptoms are present. A positive urine dipstick test for nitrites or leukocyte esterase gives an 80% probability of UTI.[18] A urine culture should be obtained if the urine dipstick testing is negative, or if symptoms fail to resolve or recur within 4 weeks of completing treatment.[4]

Postmenopausal women

Older women with acute cystitis may present a diagnostic challenge because the prevalence of chronic urinary frequency, urgency, and incontinence is higher in this population. Therefore, when considering a UTI in older women, it is important to evaluate urinary symptoms in relation to an individual's baseline.

Asymptomatic bacteriuria becomes more common with age, with a prevalence of 30% to 50% in women greater than 70 years of age,[21] which makes routine urine testing less helpful. Urine dipstick testing, urinalysis, and urine culture should not be routinely obtained in women aged 65 years or older because there is a high false-positive rate in this population.[21] Instead, in older women with a low pretest probability of UTI, urine dipstick testing can be used to rule out an infection.[22]

A diagnosis of a UTI in postmenopausal women should be made with a urine culture. Urine culture should be obtained when there are at least 2 new or worsening urinary symptoms, fever, or dysuria present for less than 1 week.[21] In patients with baseline cognitive impairment, an acute and persistent change in mental status that does not respond to the usual interventions should also prompt obtaining a urine culture.[21]

Recurrent Cystitis

The Canadian Urologic Association and European Urologic Association recommend that a diagnosis of recurrent UTI be confirmed with urine culture, at least once while symptoms are present.[4,12] A negative urine culture should prompt an investigation into other causes for the symptoms the patient is experiencing. Further investigations, such as cystoscopy or radiographic imaging with computed tomography scan of the abdomen and pelvis, should be reserved for women with risk factors for an obstruction or a structural abnormality.[4,12] The American College of Radiology Appropriateness Criteria can guide the choice of additional imaging based on the suspected abnormality (**Table 2**).[23]

Table 2
Imaging in recurrent UTIs in patients with risk factors or who do not respond to initial therapy

Suspected Abnormality	Imaging Study	ACR Recommendation
Enterovesical fistula	CT abdomen/pelvis without and with IV contrast	Usually appropriate
Pelvic organ prolapse Urethral diverticulum	MRI pelvis without and with IV contrast	May be appropriate
Pelvic organ prolapse Urinary reflux Urethral fistula	MRI without IV contrast Voiding cystourethrography CT abdomen/pelvis with IV contrast	May be appropriate
Urolithiasis	CT abdomen/pelvis without IV contrast	May be appropriate

Abbreviations: CT, computed tomography; IV, intravenous.
(*Data from* Lazarus E, Allen BC, Blaufox MD, et al. ACR Appropriateness Criteria recurrent lower urinary tract infections in women. American College of Radiology. Available at: https://acsearch.acr.org/docs/69491/Narrative. Accessed August 9, 2018.)

Uncomplicated Pyelonephritis

Urinalysis for white blood cells, red blood cells, and nitrites is recommended when a diagnosis of pyelonephritis is suspected,[4] because the results of this test are available faster than a urine culture. A urine culture and sensitivity testing are recommended for all cases of pyelonephritis.[4,6] The American College of Radiology does not recommend routine use of imaging in cases of suspected acute, uncomplicated pyelonephritis.[24] Imaging is reserved for patients who have, or are suspected of having, complicated pyelonephritis: patients with structural abnormalities, a history of recent instrumentation, indwelling urinary catheters, immunocompromised patients, and pyelonephritis in men.[9] Imaging may also be considered for patients who do not respond to appropriate antibiotic therapy within 72 hours of initiation. In these cases, a computed tomography scan of the abdomen/pelvis with intravenous (IV) contrast is recommended.[24]

Complicated Cystitis and Pyelonephritis

A urine culture should be performed for all suspected cases of complicated cystitis and pyelonephritis.[4,6] A computed tomography scan of the abdomen/pelvis with IV contrast is recommended over MRI and ultrasound examination as the imaging test of choice for complicated pyelonephritis because it is the most sensitive method for detecting urolithiasis, perinephric abscess, and emphysematous pyelonephritis.[24] Ultrasound examinations and MRI can be used in patients with contrast allergy, but they are less sensitive for small calculi and for emphysematous pyelonephritis.[24]

CLINICAL MANAGEMENT AND TREATMENT

Escherichia coli is implicated in 75% to 95% of acute uncomplicated cystitis (AUC) and pyelonephritis. Other bacteria frequently implicated in UTIs are *Proteus mirabilis*, *Klebsiella pneumonia*, and *S saprophyticus*.[6,8,12] Antibiotics are the mainstay of treatment for UTIs. The choice of antibiotic depends on the type of infection, complications, and local antimicrobial resistance patterns. The increasing antimicrobial resistance of *E coli* and the other urinary pathogens has influenced the formation of guidelines for UTI treatment[4,6] and led to the study of alternative methods of treatment for UTI.

It has been shown that 25% to 50% of women with urinary symptoms consistent with AUC recover within 1 week without antibiotics.[7] In an effort to decrease the number of antibiotic prescriptions for UTIs, a number of studies have looked at using nonsteroidal antiinflammatory drugs as a symptomatic treatment in place of antibiotics for treatment of AUC.[25–27] However, these studies have shown that nonsteroidal antiinflammatory drugs are inferior to antibiotics and, therefore, nonsteroidal antiinflammatory drugs are not recommended as a method of treatment for AUC.

Acute Uncomplicated Cystitis

There are several approaches to initiating antibiotics in women with AUC, including telephone management, patient-initiated treatment, and traditional office-visit based treatment. Telephone-based algorithms for the management of AUC have proven to be safe and cost effective, with an increase in patient satisfaction and without an increased risk of complications.[28,29] Using a telephone-based algorithm, appropriate antibiotics can be prescribed without an office visit, once risk factors for complicated infection are ruled out, and it is established that there is a high probability of infection.

Women with recurrent AUC may be managed with patient-initiated treatment.[12,30] In this method, a patient is given a prescription for an antibiotic, which can be filled when she experiences the symptoms of a UTI. If symptoms do not resolve after treatment is completed, the patient is instructed to come in for an office visit. The major risk of this method is that sexually transmitted infections such as chlamydia may be mistaken for an AUC by the patient and thus go unrecognized and untreated. Therefore, it is recommended that patient-initiated treatment not be used in women at high risk for sexually transmitted infections.[30]

When seeing a patient in the office for a suspected AUC, a delayed antibiotic approach may be used. In this method, patients are given a prescription for antibiotics, but are asked not to fill it unless they feel that they need it (eg, in cases of worsening or persistent symptoms). In a study evaluating this approach, 37% of women agreed to delay antibiotic treatment and 55% of those women improved without using antibiotics.[7] There were no complications from delaying treatment noted in this study.

Choice and duration of antibiotic

The initial antibiotic choice should be based on individual patient factors and local antibiotic resistance patterns. The current Infectious Diseases Society of America (IDSA) guidelines recommend nitrofurantoin for 5 days or trimethoprim-sulfamethoxazole (TMP-SMX) for 3 days as a first-line treatment for an AUC[6] (**Table 3**). TMP-SMX should not be used empirically in areas where known antimicrobial resistance rates are 20% or greater. A single dose of fosfomycin is also appropriate for the empiric treatment of AUC, but it may have a lower efficacy when compared with other acceptable treatments.[6,31] A 3-day course of a fluoroquinolone can be used for AUC, but to prevent the development of antimicrobial resistance, it is recommended that fluoroquinolones be reserved for more severe infections.[6]

Do not use amoxicillin or ampicillin empirically owing to high resistance rates. Cephalosporins and amoxicillin-clavulanate are less efficacious and should be not be used as empiric treatment, but can be used in 3- to 7-day regimens if other antibiotics cannot be used.[6]

Pyelonephritis

As with an AUC, the initial antibiotic choice for pyelonephritis should be based on individual patient factors and local antibiotic resistance patterns. Once the bacterial pathogen has been identified, the antibiotic regimen should be tailored appropriately.

Table 3
Treatment of AUC

Antibiotic	Dose (Oral)	Special Considerations
Nitrofurantoin monohydrate	100 mg BID ×5 d	—
TMP-SMX	160/800 mg (double strength) BID ×3 d	Not for use when resistance rates are ≥20%
Fosfomycin	3g once	—
Pivmecillinam	400 mg BID ×3–7 d	Not available in North America
Fluoroquinolones	Ciprofloxacin 250 mg BID ×3 d Ofloxacin 200 mg BID ×3 d Levofloxacin 250 mg daily ×3 d	Not recommended as a first-line agent; use only if no other agent is appropriate
Amoxicillin-clavulanate	500/125 mg BID ×3 d	Avoid unless no other agent is appropriate
Cephalosporins	Cefdinir 100 mg BID ×5 d Cefaclor 250 mg TID ×5 d Cefpodoxime-proxetil 100 mg BID ×3 d	Avoid unless no other agent is appropriate

Abbreviations: BID, 2 times per day; TID, 3 times per day.

(*Data from* Gupta K, Hooton TM, Naber KG, et al. International clinical practice guidelines for the treatment of acute uncomplicated cystitis and pyelonephritis in women: a 2010 update by the Infectious Disease Society of America and the European Society for Microbiology and Infectious Diseases. Clin Infect Dis 2011;52:e103–20.)

For outpatient treatment, the current IDSA guidelines recommend the use of an oral fluoroquinolone (ciprofloxacin or levofloxacin) as the preferred empiric therapy when local fluoroquinolone resistance rates are known to be less than 10%. If local resistance rates are 10% or greater, a one-time IV dose of ceftriaxone or another long-acting antibiotic should be given with an oral fluoroquinolone. TMP-SMX may also be used as empiric therapy with a one-time IV dose of ceftriaxone if susceptibilities are not known. Oral cephalosporins have lower efficacy compared with other agents and should only be used for the treatment of pyelonephritis if susceptibilities are known and there is no other appropriate choice. Ampicillin should only be used if infection with an *Enterococcus* is suspected owing to high resistance rates for the typical gram-negative urinary pathogens.[6]

For inpatient treatment, the IDSA recommends initiating treatment with an IV antibiotic that is appropriate based on local resistance patterns and patient factors. Fluoroquinolones, extended-spectrum penicillins, extended-spectrum cephalosporins, carbapenems, and aminoglycosides are all appropriate choices for empiric therapy.[6] The IDSA does not provide specific guidelines for when to transition to oral therapy owing to a lack of available evidence on this topic. One common practice is to choose an appropriate oral regimen once susceptibilities are available.

The duration of treatment varies based on the specific medication used (**Table 4**). With increasing antimicrobial resistance, effort should be made to use the shortest duration of antibiotics that is appropriate.[32] Fluoroquinolones have the shortest recommended length of treatment of 5 to 7 days depending on the specific drug used. The IDSA recommends that TMP-SMX be used for a total of 14 days and that beta-lactams be used for 10 to 14 days for pyelonephritis.[6] However, a metaanalysis

Table 4
Treatment of uncomplicated pyelonephritis

Antibiotic	Dose	Special Considerations
Ciprofloxacin	500 mg BID ×7 d 100 mg daily ×7 d	Can use with initial dose of Ciprofloxacin 400 mg IV Ceftriaxone 1 g IV[a]
Levofloxacin	750 mg daily ×5 d	
TMP-SMX	160/800 mg (double strength) BID ×7–14 d	Should use with initial dose of Ceftriaxone 1 g IV if susceptibilities not available

Abbreviations: BID, 2 times per day; IV, intravenous.
[a] Must be used when the prevalence of resistance to fluoroquinolones ≥10%.
(*Data from* Gupta K, Hooton TM, Naber KG, et al. International clinical practice guidelines for the treatment of acute uncomplicated cystitis and pyelonephritis in women: a 2010 update by the Infectious Disease Society of America and the European Society for Microbiology and Infectious Diseases. Clin Infect Dis 2011;52:e103–20.)

comparing the duration of treatment for pyelonephritis found that a treatment duration of 7 days or less was equivalent to a longer treatment duration and did not differ based on the type of antibiotic used.[32] Subsequently, another study comparing 7 days of TMP-SMX with 7 days of ciprofloxacin showed that the regimens were equally effective.[33] The duration of treatment does not need to be extended for patients with positive blood cultures.[32–34]

PREVENTION OF RECURRENT URINARY TRACT INFECTIONS

Both nonantimicrobial and antimicrobial prophylaxis regimens have been studied in women with recurrent UTIs (**Table 5**). With the exception of vaginal estrogen, the data supporting nonantimicrobial regimens is not robust, and additional studies are needed before routinely recommending these methods.

Vaginal Estrogen

Estrogen has a role in maintaining vaginal pH, normal vaginal flora, and urinary continence. Lower levels of estrogen in postmenopausal women are thought to be an important contributor to the higher incidence of UTIs in this population. A Cochrane review found that vaginal estrogen, used as either a cream or a ring/pessary, significantly decreased the number of UTIs in postmenopausal women.[16] Oral estrogen was not shown to decrease recurrent UTIs in postmenopausal women.[16]

Probiotics

Probiotics are thought to prevent UTIs by helping to restore the normal vaginal microbiome. A Cochrane review of 9 studies investigating the use of *Lactobacillus* spp. for the prevention of recurrent, symptomatic UTIs in women found no decrease in the risk of recurrent UTI.[35] Additional studies are needed before routinely recommending the use of probiotics to prevent recurrent UTIs.[4,12]

Cranberries

The exact mechanism by which cranberries prevent UTIs is unknown. It is thought that the proanthocyanidins found in cranberries and cranberry products inhibit *E coli* from adhering to the bladder walls. The amount of cranberry juice recommended to prevent

Table 5
Prophylaxis for recurrent UTI

Medication	Dose
Vaginal estrogen	Estradiol ring 2 mg Estradiol cream 0.5 mg nightly ×2 wk; then twice weekly
Probiotics[a]	Studied regimens include: Vaginal suppositories 2×/week to monthly Oral capsule daily to BID Oral drink 5 d/mo
Cranberries[a]	300 mL juice = 36 mg proanthocyanidins[b]
D-Mannose[a]	2 g daily
Hyaluronic acid and Chondroitin sulfate[a]	800 mg and 1 g in 50-mL solution via instillation into bladder
Antibiotics	Regimens vary May dose daily or postcoital Nitrofurantoin 50–100 mg daily TMP-SMX 40/200 daily = ½ single strength Cephalexin 125 mg daily Norfloxacin 200 mg daily

Abbreviation: BID, 2 times per day.
[a] Data are not sufficient to routinely recommend as prophylaxis.
[b] Processing of cranberries into capsules and tablets may affect the amount of proanthocyanidins they contain.
Data from Refs.[4,10,12,35–40]

UTI is 300 mL daily, an amount that many women find difficult to ingest. Capsules and tablets are better tolerated. However, the processing of cranberries may affect the amount of proanthocyanidins in cranberry tablets and capsules. A Cochrane review of 24 studies did not show any decrease in the risk of recurrent UTI in women using a variety of cranberry products.[36] Further studies are needed before routinely recommending cranberry products to prevent UTI.[4,12]

D-Mannose

One of the mechanisms by which *E coli* causes cystitis is by adhering to various proteins that line the bladder wall. D-Mannose is thought to interfere with the ability of *E coli* to bind to the urothelium. Two small studies have shown that D-mannose may be effective in preventing recurrent UTIs in women.[37,38] However, additional studies are needed before routinely recommending this method as a reliable preventive measure.

Hyaluronic Acid and Chondroitin Sulfate

The glycosaminoglycan layer lining the bladder wall, composed of hyaluronic acid and chondroitin sulfate, is thought to play a role in preventing the adherence of bacteria to the urothelium. A damaged glycosaminoglycan layer could, therefore, theoretically lead to an increased risk of recurrent UTIs. Two small, randomized, controlled trials have shown that instillation of a solution of hyaluronic acid and chondroitin sulfate can prevent recurrent UTIs.[39,40] Additional studies are needed before recommending this method as a routine preventive measure.

Antibiotics

Antibiotic prophylaxis should be reserved for those women in whom nonantimicrobial interventions have failed.[4] Various low-dose, once daily, or postcoital antibiotic regimens have been shown to be effective (see **Table 5**). A Cochrane review of antibiotic regimens for prevention of UTI showed that all studied regimens are effective in preventing UTI, and there was not enough information to conclude that one regimen was superior to another.[10] Shortly after antibiotics are discontinued, the frequency of UTIs returned to baseline level.[10]

SUMMARY

Cystitis and pyelonephritis are the most common UTIs. The classification of UTIs as complicated or uncomplicated is based on patient factors, with uncomplicated infections defined as those occurring in an otherwise healthy, nonpregnant woman with a normal genitourinary tract and no recent history of instrumentation. *Escherichia coli*, *P mirabilis*, *Klebsiella pneumoniae*, and *S saprophyticus* are the major pathogens that cause UTIs. The diagnosis and treatment of UTIs requires attention to the growing resistance of these pathogens to antibiotics. Knowledge of local antimicrobial resistance patterns is necessary when choosing an antibiotic. The most appropriate, narrowest-spectrum antibiotic should be prescribed for the shortest duration to prevent the further development of antimicrobial resistance.

REFERENCES

1. Schappert SM, Rechtsteiner EA. Ambulatory medical care utilization estimates for 2007. Vital Health Stat 13 2001;169:1–38.
2. Foxman B. Epidemiology of urinary tract infections: incidence, morbidity, and economic costs. Am J Med 2002;113:5S–13S.
3. Nicolle LE, Bradley S, Colgan R, et al. Infectious Diseases Society of America guidelines for the diagnosis and treatment of asymptomatic bacteriuria in adults. Clin Infect Dis 2005;40:643–54.
4. Bonkat G, Pickard R, Bartoletti R, et al. European Association of urology guidelines on urological infections. Available at: http://uroweb.org/guideline/urological-infections. Accessed August 7, 2018.
5. Hooton TM. Uncomplicated urinary tract infection. N Engl J Med 2012;366: 1028–37.
6. Gupta K, Hooton TM, Naber KG, et al. International clinical practice guidelines for the treatment of acute uncomplicated cystitis and pyelonephritis in women: a 2010 update by the Infectious Disease Society of America and the European Society for Microbiology and Infectious Diseases. Clin Infect Dis 2011;52:e103–20.
7. Knottnerus BJ, Geerlings SE, Moll EP, et al. Women with symptoms of uncomplicated urinary tract infection are often willing to delay antibiotic treatment: a prospective cohort study. BMC Fam Pract 2013;14:71.
8. Foxman B, Brown P. Epidemiology of urinary tract infections transmission and risk factors, incidence and costs. Infect Dis Clin North Am 2003;17:227–41.
9. Solomon CG. Acute pyelonephritis in adults. N Engl J Med 2018;378:48–59.
10. Albert X, Huertas I, Pereiro I, et al. Antibiotics for preventing recurrent urinary tract infection in non-pregnant women. Cochrane Database Syst Rev 2004;(3):CD001209.
11. Suskind AM, Saigal CS, Hanley JM, et al. Incidence and management of uncomplicated recurrent urinary tract infections in a national sample of women in the United States. Urology 2016;90:50–5.
12. Dason S, Dason JT, Kapoor A. Guidelines for the diagnosis and management of recurrent urinary tract infection in women. Can Urol Assoc J 2011;5:316–22.

13. Hooton TM, Scholes D, Hughes JP, et al. A prospective study of risk factors for symptomatic urinary tract infecction in young women. N Engl J Med 1996;335: 468–74.
14. Scholes D, Hooton TM. Risk factors for recurrent urinary tract infection in young women. J Infect Dis 2000;182:1177–82.
15. Scholes D, Hooton TM, Roberts PL, et al. Risk factors associated with acute pyelonephritis in healthy women. Ann Intern Med 2005;142:20–7.
16. Perrotta C, Aznar M, Mejia R, et al. Oestrogens for preventing recurrent urinary tract infection in postmenopausal women. Cochrane Database Syst Rev 2008;(2):CD005131.
17. Raz R, Gennesin Y, Wasser J, et al. Recurrent urinary tract infections in postmenopausal women. Clin Infect Dis 2000;30:152–6.
18. Bent S, Nallamothu BK, Simel DL, et al. Does this woman have an acute uncomplicated urinary tract infection? JAMA 2002;287:2701–10.
19. Giesen LGM, Cousins G, Dimitrov BD, et al. Predicting acute uncomplicated urinary tract infection in women: a systematic review of the diagnostic accuracy of symptoms and signs. BMC Fam Pract 2010;11:78.
20. Kranz J, Schmidt S, Lebet C, et al. The 2017 update of the German clinical guideline on epidemiology, diagnostics, therapy, prevention, and management of uncomplicated urinary tract infections in adult patients. Part II: therapy and prevention. Urol Int 2017;100:271–8.
21. Mody L, Juthani-Mehta M. Urinary tract infections in older women: a clinical review. JAMA 2014;311:844–54.
22. Devillé WL, Yzermans JC, van Duijn NP, et al. The urine dipstick test useful to rule out infections. A meta-analysis of the accuracy. BMC Urol 2004;4:4.
23. Lazarus E, Allen BC, Blaufox MD, et al. ACR Appropriateness Criteria recurrent lower urinary tract infections in women. American College of Radiology. Available at: https://acsearch.acr.org/docs/69491/Narrative. Accessed August 9, 2018.
24. Nikolaidis P, Dogra VS, Goldfardb S, et al. ACR Appropriateness Criteria acute pyelonephritis. Am Coll Radiol 2018;15(11S):S232–9. Available at: https://acsearch.acr.org/docs/69489/Narrative. Accessed August 8, 2018.
25. Gagyor I, Bleidorn J, Kochen MM, et al. Ibuprofen versus fosfomycin for uncomplicated urinary tract infection in women: randomised controlled trial. BMJ 2015; 351:h6544.
26. Kronenberg A, Butikofer L, Odutayo A, et al. Symptomatic treatment of uncomplicated lower urinary tract infections in the ambulatory setting: randomised, double blind trial. BMJ 2017;359:j4784.
27. Vik I, Bollestad M, Grude N, et al. Ibuprofen versus pivmecillinam for uncomplicated urinary tract infection in women - a double blind, randomized non-inferiority trial. PLoS Med 2018;15:e1002569.
28. Barry HC, Hickner J, Ebell MH. A randomized controlled trial of telephone management of suspected urinary tract infections in women. J Fam Pract 2001;50: 589–94.
29. Schauberger CW, Merkitch KW, Prell AM. Acute cystitis in women: experience with a telephone-based algorithm. WMJ 2007;106:326–9.
30. Gupta K, Hooton TM, Roberts PL, et al. Patient-initiated treatment of uncomplicated recurrent urinary tract infections in young women. Ann Intern Med 2001; 135:9–16.
31. Huttner A, Kowalczyk A, Turjeman A, et al. Effect of 5-day nitrofurantoin vs single-dose fosfomycin on clinical resolution of uncomplicated lower urinary tract infection in women. JAMA 2018;319:1781–9.

32. Eliakim-Raz N, Yahav D, Paul M, et al. Duration of antibiotic treatment for acute pyelonephritis and septic urinary tract infection - 7 days or less versus longer treatment: systematic review and meta-analysis of randomized controlled trials. J Antimicrob Chemother 2013;68:2183–91.
33. Fox MT, Melia MT, Same RG, et al. A seven-day course of TMP-SMX may be as effective as a seven-day course of ciprofloxacin for the treatment of pyelonephritis. Am J Med 2017;130:842–5.
34. Sandberg T, Skoog G, Bornefalk-Hermansson A, et al. Ciprofloxacin for 7 days versus 14 days in women with acute pyelonephritis: a randomised, open-label and double-blind, placebo-controlled, non-inferiority trial. Lancet 2012;380: 484–90.
35. Schwenger EM, Tejani AM, Loween PS. Probiotics for preventing urinary tract infections in adults and children. Cochrane Database Syst Rev 2015;(12):CD008772.
36. Jepson RG, Williams G, Craig JC. Cranberries for preventing urinary tract infections. Cochrane Database Syst Rev 2012;(10):CD001321.
37. Domenici L, Monti M, Bracchi C, et al. D-mannose: a promising support for acute urinary tract infections in women. A pilot study. Eur Rev Med Pharmacol Sci 2016; 20:2920–5.
38. Kranjčec B, Papeš D, Altarac S. D-mannose powder for prophylaxis of recurrent urinary tract infections in women: a randomized clinical trial. World J Urol 2014; 32:79–84.
39. Damiano R, Quarto G, Bava I, et al. Prevention of recurrent urinary tract infections by intravesical administration of hyaluronic acid and chondroitin sulphate: a placebo-controlled randomised trial. Eur Urol 2011;59:645–51.
40. De Vita D, Giordano S. Effectiveness of intravesical hyaluronic acid/chondroitin sulfate in recurrent bacterial cystitis: a randomized study. Int Urogynecol J 2012;23:1707–13.

Nephrolithiasis

Laura Mayans, MD, MPH

KEYWORDS

• Nephrolithiasis • Kidney stones • Dual-energy flank pain

KEY POINTS

- Nephrolithiasis was a common ancient disease and remains a significant source of morbidity and medical expenditure today.
- Nephrolithiasis presents as acute flank or abdominal pain with nausea and vomiting. Hematuria is present in 90% of cases, but its absence does not rule out nephrolithiasis.
- Noncontrasted computed tomography scan is first-line to diagnose kidney stones in nonpregnant adults. Ultrasound is first-line in children and pregnant women.
- Most cases can be managed expectantly as an outpatient with hydration, analgesia, and possibly medications to aide in passage.
- A metabolic evaluation may be indicated after a second episode of nephrolithiasis in adults or after a first episode in children or those with a family history of nephrolithiasis.

INTRODUCTION

Nephrolithiasis is an acutely painful, often recurrent, condition that affects all ages, races, and genders. Descriptions of nephrolithiasis can be found in ancient texts of the Indians, Chinese, and Greeks.[1] The Hippocratic Oath even references stone disease.[1] It remains a common disease in the United States and around the world. Prevalence of nephrolithiasis in increasing and with it medical expenditure. The total cost associated with kidney stones rose by 50% between 1994 and 2000, despite a shift from inpatient to outpatient management.[1] Nephrolithiasis is a common condition with significant associated morbidity and cost to society.

EPIDEMIOLOGY

The prevalence of nephrolithiasis in the United States has increased 70% in the past 30 years.[2] According to the 2010 National Health and Nutrition Examination Survey (NHANES) study, kidney stone prevalence was 10.6% in men and 7.1% in women, with an overall prevalence of 8.8% (vs 5.2% in the 1988–1994 NHANES study).[2]

Disclosure: The author has nothing to disclose.
Department of Family and Community Medicine, University of Kansas School of Medicine – Wichita, Hillside Medical Office 855 N. Hillside Wichita, KS 67214, USA
E-mail address: lmayans@kumc.edu

Prim Care Clin Office Pract 46 (2019) 203–212
https://doi.org/10.1016/j.pop.2019.02.001

This increase has occurred across all ages, races, and genders.[2,3] The greatest increases occurred in the black, non-Hispanic population and in women.[1,3]

Kidney stone incidence varies by sex, racial background, geography, and age in the United States. It is most common in white male individuals and least common in black female individuals.[1,4,5] Prevalence is highest in the southeastern United States.[1,4] In male individuals, kidney stone incidence begins to rise after age 20 and peaks between 40 and 60.[4] In female individuals, incidence peaks much earlier: in the late 20s.[4]

Kidney stone prevalence is increasing globally as well. Studies report rising rates in Germany, Italy, Japan, Spain, Greece, and Turkey.[1,5] Stone composition differs between developed and developing countries, likely related to dietary differences.[1,5] Calcium-containing stones are more common in developed countries.[1]

RISK FACTORS AND ASSOCIATIONS

There is an absence of large, randomized controlled trials in kidney stone disease. In addition to NHANES data, 3 large cohort studies have been used to investigate risk factors for nephrolithiasis occurrence and recurrence.[2] These studies are the Nurse's Health Study I, Nurse's Health Study II, and the Health Professionals Follow-up Study. All 3 studies found associations between nephrolithiasis and weight gain, body mass index (BMI), and diabetes mellitus.[3] Both a higher baseline BMI and a 35 pound or more weight gain since early adulthood significantly increased the risk of developing a kidney stone, and the increased risk was greater in women than men.[1,3] A history of type 2 diabetes mellitus also increased risk for kidney stone development, independent of diet and body size. Several other nondietary risk factors exist[2,4]:

- Family history: a family history of kidney stones increases risk by 2.5 times
- Systemic disease: primary hyperparathyroidism, renal tubular acidosis, and Crohn disease increase risk
- History of gout: increases the likelihood of forming both uric acid stones and calcium stones
- Working (or living) in a hot environment

Urine composition is influenced by dietary composition, and the high or low intake of several nutrients are linked to an increased risk of kidney stone formation.[2,4] High urinary excretion of substances such as calcium, oxalate, cysteine, and uric acid promote stone formation, whereas substances like citrate and magnesium are protective.[4] Most stones in the United States are calcium-containing; however, high dietary calcium intake actually lowers kidney stone risk. This may be because high calcium intake decreases oxalate absorption and urinary excretion, or there may be other protective factors in dairy products, which is the primary source of dietary calcium in the United States.[4] Although inconsistent, some studies show increased risk of kidney stones in those who take calcium supplements, especially older women.[4] Although some still question whether high dietary calcium is protective, most agree that calcium *restriction* is not beneficial, and could be harmful, especially in terms of bone health.

The most common type of kidney stone is a calcium oxalate stone.[6] However, the role of dietary oxalate in kidney stone formation is unclear and controversial. High-quality studies of its impact are lacking, but may be possible in the future.[4]

Fluid intake is an important modifiable risk factor for kidney stones.[1,2,4] High fluid intake consistently appears protective, whereas low fluid intake increases risk. It does not appear to matter what fluid is consumed. Only grapefruit juice was shown to increase risk, and milk consumption appears to lower risk. Coffee, tea, beer, wine, and orange juice had no significant effect on kidney stone formation.[4] Consumption of soda (with/without caffeine, sugared or diet) and risk of kidney stones is less clear and studies disagree. Some find sugar-sweetened beverages increase risk; others find no association.[2,4,5]

The effects of other studied nutrients vary by age, sex, and BMI.[4] High animal protein intake may increase risk in normal-weight men. Sucrose may increase risk in women. Potassium and magnesium supplementation may lower risk in men, but not in women. High vitamin C supplementation can increase risk in those known to form calcium oxalate stones. Dietary vitamin C should not be restricted, but vitamin C supplementation should be discouraged.[4] High intake of fruits, fiber, and vegetables lowers risk in women.[1]

Of note, nephrolithiasis has been found to be a risk factor for the future development of hypertension, cardiovascular disease, and chronic kidney disease, although the associations are weaker and differ between men and women.[6] Several components of the metabolic syndrome are more common in those who form kidney stones than in those who do not. In addition to overweight/obesity and diabetes, higher cholesterol and triglyceride levels also can be seen.[6] Causality, however, cannot be established by studies to date.

CLINICAL PRESENTATION

The most common presenting symptoms of nephrolithiasis are sudden-onset, crampy flank pain, hematuria, nausea, and vomiting.[7–9] The pain waxes and wanes in the acute phase and patients are often unable to find a comfortable position and appear writhing in pain.[8] Although often described as excruciating, the pain also can be a dull pressure or dragging sensation.[9] Constant pain at the onset raises concern of a more severe obstruction.[7] Early on, the pain often radiates to the groin.[8] As the stone descends, the pain may localize to the abdomen. As it approaches the vesicoureteral junction, pain can be felt at the tip of the urethra, causing dysuria and a persistent urge to urinate.[8,9] Pain with palpation of the costovertebral angle and/or lower quadrant are common.[8]

Approximately 50% of patients present with nausea and vomiting, resulting from shared splanchnic innervation of the renal capsule and intestines.[7,8] Hematuria, either macroscopic or microscopic, is present in nearly 90% of cases, but the absence of hematuria does not rule out stone disease.[7–9] More than 10% of proven stone passages have been found to present without hematuria.[9]

Fever and chills at presentation are unusual and suggest the presence of an infected stone or concurrent urinary tract infection (UTI).[7] Tachycardia and hypertension can be seen and are usually secondary to pain.[7]

It is important to note that elderly individuals are more likely to have atypical presentations.[7] In one study involving more than 1500 symptomatic stone formers, increasing age was associated with a greater likelihood of presenting with atypical or no pain, fever, gastrointestinal symptoms, pyuria, and UTI.[10] Increasing age was also associated with larger stone diameter and increased need for surgical intervention.

DIAGNOSIS

A few routine laboratory tests are indicated in the workup of acute flank pain, but definitive diagnosis of nephrolithiasis is achieved through imaging. Initial laboratory testing involves urinalysis and serum chemistry to evaluate hematuria and creatinine clearance.[7] A complete blood count with differential is reasonable if the patient presents with systemic signs of infection or an alternate abdominal etiology is strongly suspected. A woman of reproductive age should receive a pregnancy test. Microscopic hematuria is present in more than 90% of cases.[7] Pyuria is also often present, but not necessarily indicative of concurrent infection. The stone itself can cause ureteral inflammation, resulting in white blood cells (WBCs) on urinalysis.[7] The greater the degree of pyuria, the greater the likelihood of infection. More than 50 WBCs per high-power field is associated with a 60% culture-positive rate.[7] The presence of leukocyte esterase or nitrites also increases the likelihood of a concurrent UTI.

Multiple imaging modalities are available for the diagnosis of nephrolithiasis, including plain-film KUB (kidney, ureter, bladder), ultrasonography, computed tomography (CT), and MRI. Intravenous pyelogram was historically used but has essentially been replaced by CT.[11] Each imaging modality has distinct advantages and disadvantages, and some are more appropriate in special circumstances. **Table 1** lists the common imaging modalities and their sensitivities and specificities for the detection of kidney stones.

Most stones are calcium containing, and are therefore radiopaque. Yet plain-film KUB has the lowest sensitivity and specificity of all available modalities.[7,11] Identification of stones can be hindered by body habitus, overlying bowel gas, and extrarenal calcifications. It is also unable to evaluate for hydronephrosis or exact stone location.

Noncontrasted CT scan of the abdomen and pelvis is the gold standard for the diagnosis of nephrolithiasis in the United States.[7,9,11,12] CT scan can detect all stone types, specifically locate them within the urinary system, and allows for measurement of the stone, to aide in prognosis.[7,11,12] It can identify for hydronephrosis as well as alternate causes for the patient's pain if the scan is negative for a stone.[7,12] The primary disadvantage of CT is the radiation exposure. Low-dose CT scan protocols have been studied and low-dose CT scan shows comparable sensitivity and specificity, but can miss small stones (<2–3 mm) and stones in obese patients.[7,11]

Ultrasonography for the diagnosis of kidney stones is increasingly used worldwide, including in the United States.[7,9,12] Advantages are its lack of radiation exposure, relative low cost, and ease of use. In many parts of the world, ultrasound machines are much more widely available than CT scanners. In the United States it is still considered second-line to CT. However, it is the first-line imaging modality for children and pregnant women, in whom radiation exposure is most dangerous.[7,9,11,12] Ultrasound indirectly detects stones by identifying hydronephrosis.[7,12] Stones can be directly visualized as hyperechoic lines with distal shadowing. Adding color Doppler allows visualization of the "twinkling sign," which is alternating colors deep to the visualized stone.[7] Ultrasound can be limited by user experience as well as body habitus.[11] A 2014 studied examined ultrasonography versus CT for suspected nephrolithiasis.[13]

Table 1
Sensitivity, specificity, and American College of Radiology rating for common imaging modalities

Imaging Modality	Sensitivity, %	Specificity, %
KUB	45–58	60–77
Ultrasonography	54–64	91–100
CT	91–100	95–100
MRI	NR	~93

Abbreviations: CT, computed tomography; KUB, kidney, ureter, bladder; NR, not reported.
Data from Refs.[7,9,11]

Table 2
STONE score

Criteria	Points
Sex	
Male	2
Female	0
Timing (when did pain start)	
<6 h prior	3
6–24 h prior	1
>24 h prior	0
Origin (ethnicity)	
Non-black	3
Black	0
Nausea	
Vomiting alone	2
Nausea alone	1
None	0
Erythrocytes (hematuria on urinalysis)	
Present	3
Absent	0
Total points possible	13

From Gottlieb M, Long B, Koyfman A. The evaluation and management of urolithiasis in the ED: a review of the literature. Am J Emerg Med 2018;36(4):702; with permission.

Although ultrasound sensitivity and specificity were lower, there were no significant differences in outcomes between the groups, including complications, serious adverse events, pain scores, return emergency department visits, or hospitalizations.[13] This may suggest that the stones missed by ultrasound are not likely to be of clinical significance and are likely to pass spontaneously.

MRI does not directly visualize stones but instead relies on calcifications and signal voids. It is costly, time-consuming, and not readily available in many cases.[11] For those reasons, it is of very low utility in the evaluation of suspected nephrolithiasis. Its primary use is in pregnant women with suspected nephrolithiasis when ultrasound is nondiagnostic.[7,11]

A validated risk assessment tool was derived and validated by Moore and colleagues in 2014.[14] Titled the STONE Criteria, it uses 5 criteria (sex, timing, origin, nausea, and erythrocytes on urinalysis) to place patients into low, moderate, or high probability of having a stone in the ureter. Scoring is shown in **Table 2**. **Table 3** shows derived and validated likelihoods for each group. Subsequent external validations demonstrated a prevalence of 13.5% to 21.8% in the low-probability group, 32.3% to 80.1% in the moderate-probability group, and 72.7% to 98.7% in the high-probability group.[7] Others have modified the criteria to include C-reactive protein or ultrasound examination findings, but both modified tools require further validation. The STONE tool may help defer CT imaging in some patients.

MANAGEMENT

Analgesia is the first step in management of nephrolithiasis.[7,8] Nonsteroidal anti-inflammatory drugs (NSAIDs) and/or narcotics are traditionally used. The direct effects

Table 3
Derivation and validation of the STONE risk assessment tool

Score	Derived Likelihood, %	Validated Likelihood, %
Low probability (score 0–5)	8.3	9.2
Moderate probability (score 6–9)	51.6	51.3
High probability (score 10–13)	89.6	88.6

Abbreviation: STONE, sex, timing, origin, nausea, and erythrocytes on urinalysis.

Data from Gottlieb M, Long B, Koyfman A. The evaluation and management of urolithiasis in the ED: A review of the literature. Am J Emerg Med 2018;36(4):699–706; and Moore CL, Bomann S, Daniels B, et al. Derivation and validations of a clinical prediction rule for uncomplicated ureteral stone – the STONE score: retrospective and prospective observational cohort studies. BMJ 2014; 348:g2191.

of NSAIDs on prostaglandins and inflammation decrease smooth muscle stimulation and ureteral spasm. They are most effective if administered intravenously.[8] Although there is a theoretic worry for worsened renal function or increased bleeding if a surgical procedure becomes necessary, studies have shown that common doses of ketorolac pose little to no increased risk of renal deterioration or increased bleeding.[8] If NSAIDs are ineffective at relieving acute pain, use of opioid narcotics is reasonable.[7,8,15] Intravenous (IV) fluids have often been used with the intention of flushing out stones; however studies do not support this practice. IV fluids should be used to treat dehydration; not used solely for stone expulsion.

The clinician must also determine if urgent intervention is required. Signs that warrant hospitalization and urgent urology consultation include an obstructed and infected upper urinary system, intractable pain or vomiting, anuria, or any high-grade obstruction of a transplanted or solitary kidney.[8,15] If urgent intervention is not indicated, expectant management as an outpatient is appropriate in most situations. Stone size is the best predictor of spontaneous passage. Most stones <5 mm in diameter pass spontaneously. **Table 4** lists stone sizes and rates of spontaneous passage.

Two-thirds of kidney stones pass spontaneously within 4 weeks.[15] For this reason, an observation period of 2 to 4 weeks is reasonable. The use of alpha-adrenergic

Table 4
Stone size and passage rate

Stone Size, mm	Mean Days to Passage	Passage Rate, %[a]
1 2	8	87
3	12	76
4 5 6	22	60
7 8–9 >9	NR	48 25

[a] The reported likelihood of needing intervention was 3% for stones <2 mm, 50% for stones measuring 4–6 mm, and 99% for stones >6 mm.

Data from Gottlieb M, Long B, Koyfman A. The evaluation and management of urolithiasis in the ED: A review of the literature. Am J Emerg Med 2018;36(4):699–706; and AUAUniversity. Medical student curriculum: kidney stones. Available at: http://www.auanet.org/education/auauniversity/medical-student-education/medical-student-curriculum/kidney-stones. Accessed June 7, 2018.

medications, such as tamsulosin, which relax urinary smooth muscle, have been shown to increase stone passage rate.[7] Known as medical expulsive therapy or MET, it also decreases the time of stone passage as well as the need for pain medication.[7,15] MET is most effective for small stones in the distal ureter.[15] Stones larger than 5 mm or stones that have not moved or passed within 1 month warrant referral to urology for consideration of lithotripsy or surgical intervention.[7,8,15]

First-time stone formers should be encouraged to strain their urine to catch the stone so it may be submitted for analysis. Knowledge of stone composition can have implications for management of future stone episodes, as well as suggest possible dietary or lifestyle changes for prevention. For instance, uric acid stones can be fully managed medically. Uric acid stones are dissolved by alkalinizing the patient's urine with potassium citrate.[8,15]

The need for metabolic testing in people who form kidney stones is debated. Approximately 50% of stone formers will experience recurrence within 10 years.[7,8] Not all risk factors are controllable, but when identified, specific dietary changes can decrease the risk of recurrence. Still, the impact of testing on outcomes is not clear, as the long-term adherence to recommended changes can be as low as 30%.[8] The American Urologic Association recommends a metabolic evaluation in recurrent stone formers as well as initial stone formers believed to be at high risk for recurrence, such as those with a positive family history of kidney stones, pediatric patients, and young adults (Grade B recommendation).[2]

A standard metabolic evaluation includes an analysis of stone composition and two 24-hour urine collections, examined for total volume, pH, calcium, oxalate, uric acid, citrate, sodium, potassium, and creatinine.[2,15] Experts also recommend checking serum calcium, phosphorous, uric acid, bicarbonate, blood urea nitrogen, creatinine, albumin, alkaline phosphatase, and if calcium is high or hyperparathyroidism is suspected, intact parathyroid hormone and 1,25-dihydroxyvitamin D.[15] The most common identified abnormalities are low urine volume, hypercalciuria, hyperoxaluria, hypocitraturia, and hyperuricosuria.[15]

General beneficial dietary changes include decreasing sodium and animal protein intake, maintaining adequate calcium intake, increasing water consumption (to generate a urine volume of 2.0–2.5 L/d), and increasing consumption of fruits and vegetables.[2,7,15] Specific metabolic abnormalities can benefit from specific dietary changes. A listing can be found at http://www.auanet.org/guidelines/medical-management-of-kidney-stones-(2014).

Some medications can be offered to *recurrent* stone formers.[2] For recurrent calcium-containing stones, thiazide diuretics can be used in those found to have an increased urinary calcium, whereas potassium citrate is useful in those found to have low or low normal urine citrate. Both medications can be considered in calcium stone formers who have no identified abnormality, yet form recurrent stones. Calcium oxalate stone formers with an increased urinary uric acid and normal urine calcium can benefit from allopurinol. Uric acid and cystine stone formers can be given potassium citrate therapy to increase the pH of their urine. It is NOT advised to routinely offer allopurinol to all uric acid stone formers.

SPECIAL POPULATIONS

Pediatrics

As opposed to adults, in children, girls are more likely to develop nephrolithiasis. Overall incidence is lower in children but has been increasing over the past 25 years.[1,16] Prevalence increased threefold between 1999 and 2007.[16] This rapid increase suggests an environmental cause, with dietary change and its associated increase in obesity as the most favored etiology.[1,16,17] The increased availability of fast and processed foods has led to an increase in sodium, animal protein, and carbohydrate consumption and decreased water consumption, all of which increase the risk of stone formation.[1,16,17] The rise in prevalence of nephrolithiasis in children parallels the rise in pediatric obesity.[1,17] Calcium oxalate stones account for 60% to 90% of stones in children, followed by calcium phosphate stones.[17]

Children with nephrolithiasis present similarly to adults, with flank and/or abdominal pain and hematuria. The diagnostic workup is similar to that of adults. Initial workup includes urinalysis and imaging. Although CT scan is first-line in adults, ultrasound is the preferred first-line imaging modality in children because of concerns about radiation exposure.[16] Management mirrors that of adults. Analgesia is the first step, and narcotics are often required.[16] The need for urgent consultation should be determined using the factors as for adults. A child may need to be hospitalized if he or she requires IV analgesia, IV fluids, or displays signs or symptoms of concurrent infection.[16] Otherwise children can be managed expectantly as an outpatient. Stones <4 mm are likely to spontaneously pass in children of all ages.[16] Stones >5 mm are likely to require intervention, such as lithotripsy, stent placement, or ureteroscopy.[16] MET with alpha-adrenergic blockers or calcium channel blocks has been used in older children, although studies supporting this practice are few.[16] An attempt to catch the stone should be made because stone analysis is even more important in children, because they are more likely to have recurrence.[16]

More than 50% of children with nephrolithiasis will be found to have an underlying metabolic disorder. Therefore a metabolic workup is recommended after the first stone event in all children. The workup is the same as for adults and includes stone analysis and 24-hour urine collection and analysis. The commonly encountered abnormalities include high urinary calcium, oxalate, uric acid, or cystine and decreased urinary citrate or magnesium.[16] Prevention is based on the results of the metabolic workup with dietary changes for children identical to that recommended for adults. All children should be encouraged to increase fluid intake, decrease sodium consumption, and maintain adequate calcium consumption.[16] Low calcium intake will cause the intestines to absorb more oxalate, leading to increased risk of calcium oxalate stones.[17] Thiazide diuretics and potassium citrate can also be used in children for the same indications as in adults.[16]

Pregnant Women

Acute abdominal pain in an obstetric patient is considered an emergency and obstetric causes must be ruled out first. Nephrolithiasis is the most common nonobstetric cause of acute abdominal pain during pregnancy.[12] Diagnosis and treatment of nephrolithiasis in pregnancy is challenging because of the effects of imaging and medications on the developing fetus.

Normal anatomic and physiologic changes of pregnancy can promote stone formation and also complicate diagnosis and management. During pregnancy the upper urinary tract dilates, likely from the effects of progesterone on smooth muscle as well as pressure on the ureters from the gravid uterus.[18–20] This is seen as early as the seventh week in 90% of pregnant women and can last up to 6 weeks postpartum.[20] This leads to urinary stasis, which can predispose pregnant women to nephrolithiasis, as well as UTIs and pyelonephritis.[12,20] Still, the rate of nephrolithiasis in pregnant women is similar to that of age-matched controls.[18,19] This is likely because pregnancy is associated with increased urinary excretion of both stone-promoting substances like calcium and uric acid, as well as stone-inhibiting substances like citrate and magnesium.[18] Nephrolithiasis is most common in the second and third trimesters when anatomic changes within the abdomen due to the expanding gravid uterus can alter the location and radiation of pain.[19] A high index of suspicion for nephrolithiasis is indicated when obstetric causes of abdominal pain have been ruled out.

Limited imaging options make definitive diagnosis challenging. Ultrasound is the recommended first-line modality, as it lacks radiation and poses negligible risk to the fetus.[12,19,20] However, as stated previously, a degree of hydronephrosis is normal in pregnancy, which makes interpretation difficult if stones are not directly visualized.[20] The sensitivity and specificity improve when the degree of hydronephrosis is compared with that on the unaffected side and when color Doppler is used to evaluate for the "twinkling sign" and presence of ureteral jets into the bladder.[20] MRI is considered second-line, as it is less available, more expensive, and cannot directly visualize stones. In rare situations, low-dose CT scanning has been used.[12,19,20] Determining stone size can be very difficult in pregnancy because of imaging limitations.

Conservative management is first-line whenever possible. This includes bed rest, hydration, and analgesia. Women may need to be hospitalized for IV hydration, analgesia, and fetal monitoring.[19,20] The safety of MET using alpha-adrenergics or calcium channel blockers has not been studied.[20] Passage rates of stones during pregnancy appear to be as good as or better than rates in nonpregnant women, with studies reporting spontaneous passage rates of 64% to 70%.[19,20] Fifty percent of remaining patients will pass the stone in the postpartum period.[20]

When intervention is required, options are also limited. Procedures that do not require general anesthesia, use of ionizing radiation, or prone positioning are preferred. Percutaneous drainage and stenting or ureteroscopy are the best options.[19,20] Lithotripsy is contraindicated in pregnancy.[19,20]

A retrospective study conducted in 1989 to 2010 examined the association between nephrolithiasis in pregnancy and multiple patient characteristics and pregnancy outcomes.[18] Existing obesity and hypertensive disorders were independent risk factors for developing kidney stones. Those who developed kidney stones had higher rates of subsequent hypertensive disorders, gestational diabetes, and cesarean deliveries. This study found no increased risk of adverse perinatal outcomes, including premature rupture of the membranes, preterm delivery, low birth weight or APGAR scores, or perinatal mortality. However, other studies have seen a slight increase in preterm labor in women with nephrolithiasis in pregnancy.[19]

Anatomic Abnormalities

Anyone with known abnormal urinary tracts are at increased risk of complications from nephrolithiasis. Such abnormalities could include transplanted kidneys, solitary kidneys, horseshoe kidneys, polycystic kidney disease, or urinary diversions. Although diagnosis is often similar in these patients, management is best coordinated by urologic specialists, who should be consulted quickly after diagnosis of kidney stones.[19]

COMING ADVANCEMENTS

The biggest developing advancement in the management of nephrolithiasis is the availability and use of dual-energy CT (DECT) scanners.[12] DECT has the potential to differentiate between stone types and create a virtual, unenhanced image of the stone. Different stone types exhibit different attenuation values, which can be compared with known values and stone composition determined.[12] This is done using less radiation than standard CT scanners and can result in quicker, more directed treatment of kidney stones.[12]

As CT scan technology improves and can be performed with lower and lower doses of radiation, it may gain increasing favor for use in pediatric patients, or possibly pregnant patients in certain situations. However, much further research is needed to establish safety.

REFERENCES

1. Shoag J, Tasian GE, Goldfarb DS, et al. The new epidemiology of nephrolithiasis. Adv Chronic Kidney Dis 2015;22(4):273–8.
2. American Urological Association Medical Management of Kidney Stones Guidelines. Available at: http://www.auanet.org/guidelines/medical-management-of-kidney-stones-(2014). Accessed May 22, 2018.
3. Scales CD, Smith AC, Hanley JM, et al. Prevalence of kidney stones in the United States. Eur Urol 2012;62(1):160–5.
4. Curhan GC. Epidemiology of stone disease. Urol Clin North Am 2007;34(3):287–93.
5. Romero V, Akpinar H, Assimos DG. Kidney stones: a global picture of prevalence, incidence, and associated risk factors. Rev Urol 2010;12(2/3):e86–96.
6. Inci M, Demirtas A, Sarli B, et al. Association between body mass index, lipid profiles, and types of urinary stones. Ren Fail 2012;34(9):1140–3.
7. Gottlieb M, Long B, Koyfman A. The evaluation and management of urolithiasis in the ED: a review of the literature. Am J Emerg Med 2018;36(4):699–706.
8. Teichman JMH. Acute renal colic from ureteral calculus. N Engl J Med 2004;350(7):684–93.
9. Pfau A, Knauf F. Update on nephrolithiasis: core curriculum 2016. Am J Kidney Dis 2016;68(6):973–85.
10. Krambeck AE, Lieske JC, Xujian L, et al. Effect of age on the clinical presentation of incident symptomatic urolithiasis in the general population. J Urol 2013;189:158–64.
11. Mandeville JA, Gnessin E, Lingeman JE. Imaging evaluation in the patient with renal stone disease. Semin Nephrol 2011;31(3):254–8.
12. McCarthy CJ, Baliyan V, Kordbacheh H, et al. Radiology of renal stone disease. Int J Surg 2016;36:638–46.
13. Smith-Bindman R, Aubin C, Bailitz J, et al. Ultrasonography versus computed tomography for suspected nephrolithiasis. N Engl J Med 2014;371(12):1100–10.
14. Moore CL, Bomann S, Daniels B, et al. Derivation and validations of a clinical prediction rule for uncomplicated ureteral stone – the STONE score: retrospective and prospective observational cohort studies. BMJ 2014;348:g2191.
15. AUAUniversity. Medical Student Curriculum: Kidney Stones. Available at: http://www.auanet.org/education/auauniversity/medical-student-education/medical-student-curriculum/kidney-stones. Accessed June 7, 2018.
16. Valentini RP, Lakshmanan Y. Nephrolithiasis in children. Adv Chronic Kidney Dis 2011;18(5):370–5.
17. Lopez M, Hoppe B. History, epidemiology, and regional diversities of urolithiasis. Pediatr Nephrol 2010;25:49–59.
18. Rosenberg E, Sergienko R, Abu-Ghanem S, et al. Nephrolithiasis during pregnancy: characteristics, complications, and pregnancy outcome. World J Urol 2011;29:743–7.
19. Tan Y, Cha DY, Gupta M. Management of stones in abnormal situations. Urol Clin North Am 2013;40:79–97.
20. Thomas AA, Thomas AZ, Campbell SC, et al. Urologic emergencies in pregnancy. Pediatr Urol 2010;76(2):453–60.

Bladder Pain Syndrome

Check for updates

Miranda M. Huffman, MD, MEd[a,*], Aniesa Slack, MD[b], Maris Hoke, MD[b]

KEYWORDS

- Interstitial cystitis • Bladder pain syndrome • Painful bladder syndrome
- Chronic pelvic pain

KEY POINTS

- Bladder pain syndrome (also known as interstitial cystitis) is an unpleasant sensation that the patient attributes to the bladder, with other lower urinary symptoms that are not attributable to another cause.
- History, physical examination, and urinalysis are generally sufficient to rule out other causes; cystoscopy is not necessary to confirm the diagnosis.
- All patients with BPS should be counseled on avoiding dietary triggers and managing the symptoms with bladder retraining, hydration, and stress management.
- Oral treatments should be directed at the patient's specific symptoms.
- Pelvic floor physical therapy should be considered in most patients.

INTRODUCTION

Bladder pain syndrome (BPS), also known as painful bladder syndrome or interstitial cystitis, is one cause of chronic pelvic pain.[1,2] It is part of the spectrum of chronic pelvic pain syndromes and often co-exists with other conditions (eg, endometriosis, chronic prostatitis, irritable bowel syndrome, vaginismus, fibromyalgia).[3–5] Traditionally the diagnosis required cystoscopy; however, relying on pathognomonic findings on cystoscopy results in underdiagnosis of the common condition. Cystoscopy can be considered to rule out other conditions or to initiate treatments.[1]

PATHOGENESIS AND RISK FACTORS

Variations in diagnostic criteria have made it difficult to determine epidemiology; the largest study in the United States reports a prevalence between 2.7% and 6.5% of women.[6] Studies have shown a female-to-male preponderance of 5:1.[7] The precise cause of BPS is not known, but is likely multifactorial and varies from patient

Disclosure: The authors have nothing to disclose.
[a] Department of Family and Community Medicine, Meharry Medical College, 1005 Dr. DB Todd Jr Boulevard, Nashville, TN 37208, USA; [b] Department of Community and Family Medicine, University of Missouri-Kansas City, 7900 Lee's Summit Road, Kansas City, MO 64139-1236, USA
* Corresponding author.
E-mail address: MHuffman@mmc.edu

Prim Care Clin Office Pract 46 (2019) 213–221
https://doi.org/10.1016/j.pop.2019.02.002

to patient. Possible causes include chronic systemic inflammation, subclinical infection, urothelial dysfunction, autoimmunity, genetics, and dysfunction in central pain processing.[8–10]

DIAGNOSIS

Patients usually present in the third or fourth decade of life with recurrent episodes of urinary frequency, urgency, and nocturia associated with bladder pain or pressure (**Box 1**). The pain or pressure typically increases with increased bladder volume. Although patients with overactive bladder syndrome generally void to avoid incontinence, patients with BPS void to relieve pain. The location of pain in BPS is usually suprapubic but sometimes radiates to the groin, vagina, rectum, and sacrum, and dyspareunia is reported in up to 60% of young patients. Therefore, any patient with chronic pelvic pain should be asked specifically about pain with bladder filling, nocturia, and frequency.[1,2,5,8] Patients may have been treated for acute cystitis multiple times in the past with normal urinalysis or negative urine cultures.

Initial evaluation should focus on ruling out other causes of the patient's symptoms (**Table 1**). This generally requires a complete history, physical examination including pelvic examination in women and rectal examination in men, and urinalysis.[1,11] Cystoscopy is not required for diagnosis, although it is often performed during the work-up to exclude other causes for bladder pain, and can be helpful in the identification of Hunner's lesions. Hunner's lesions are circumscript, reddened mucosal areas and are associated with more severe symptoms and smaller bladder capacity. Their identification may help direct treatment strategies, as discussed later.[2,12]

Bladder cancer should be considered in patients with hematuria or other risk factors (older patients, tobacco exposure, occupational exposures), and such patients should be referred for cystoscopy.[13,14]

MANAGEMENT APPROACH

Once the diagnosis is confirmed based on symptoms, and other diseases are ruled out, management should focus on patient education, avoiding catastrophizing, and maximizing function.[1,15,16] Counseling patients on the course of the disease and expected outcomes of treatment is paramount.[1] There is no curative treatment, but symptoms can be managed to improve quality of life.[2] There is a strong placebo effect in BPS.[17]

Key principles of management of bladder pain syndrome:

1. Focus on maximizing function
2. Target interventions to the patient's specific symptoms (guidelines refer to this as *phenotype-directed therapy*)[2]
3. Use a stepwise approach from most conservative to most invasive (**Fig. 1** for a summary of this approach)[1,2]

Box 1
Diagnostic criteria for bladder pain syndrome

1. Unpleasant symptoms the patient attributes to the bladder
2. Other lower urinary symptoms (eg, urinary frequency)
3. Present for at least 6 weeks
4. No other cause of symptoms

Table 1
Other diagnoses to consider

Other Diagnoses to Consider	Tests to Consider
Urinary tract infection	Urinalysis Urine culture
Bladder or ureteral calculi	CT abdomen and pelvis without contrast
Genital herpes	Genital examination
Vaginitis, urethritis	Chlamydia and gonorrhea PCR Wet mount
Urinary retention	Post-void residual Urodynamics
Bladder cancer	Cystoscopy
Cervical, uterine, or ovarian cancer	Pelvic examination Pap smear Pelvic ultrasound
Endometriosis	Pelvic examination Diagnostic laparoscopy
Prostatitis	Rectal examination PSA

Abbreviations: CT, computed tomography; PCR, polymerase chain reaction; PSA, prostrate-specific antigen.

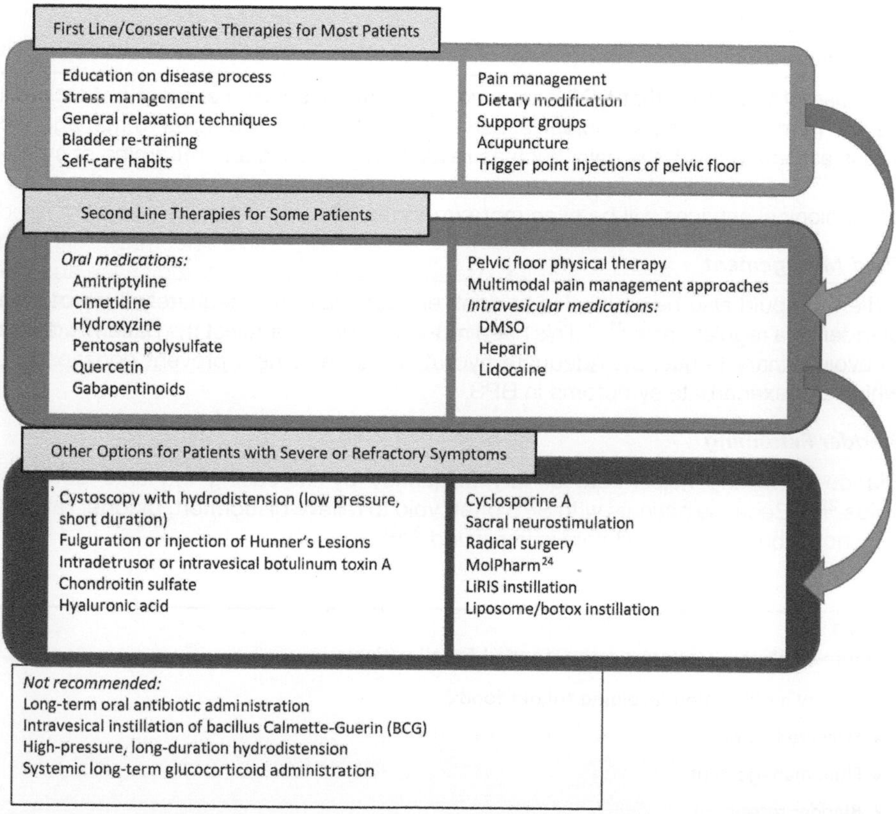
First Line/Conservative Therapies for Most Patients
Education on disease process
Stress management
General relaxation techniques
Bladder re-training
Self-care habits
Pain management
Dietary modification
Support groups
Acupuncture
Trigger point injections of pelvic floor
Second Line Therapies for Some Patients
Oral medications:
Amitriptyline
Cimetidine
Hydroxyzine
Pentosan polysulfate
Quercetin
Gabapentinoids
Pelvic floor physical therapy
Multimodal pain management approaches
Intravesicular medications:
DMSO
Heparin
Lidocaine
Other Options for Patients with Severe or Refractory Symptoms
Cystoscopy with hydrodistension (low pressure, short duration)
Fulguration or injection of Hunner's Lesions
Intradetrusor or intravesical botulinum toxin A
Chondroitin sulfate
Hyaluronic acid
Cyclosporine A
Sacral neurostimulation
Radical surgery
MolPharm[24]
LiRIS instillation
Liposome/botox instillation
Not recommended:
Long-term oral antibiotic administration
Intravesical instillation of bacillus Calmette-Guerin (BCG)
High-pressure, long-duration hydrodistension
Systemic long-term glucocorticoid administration

Fig. 1. Stepwise approach from most conservative to most invasive.

4. If severe symptoms, consider starting multiple treatments simultaneously[1,2,18]
5. Ineffective treatments should be stopped after a reasonable therapeutic trial[1]

Pain control, both pharmacologic and non-pharmacologic, should be part of the treatment plan and managed like other chronic pain conditions, including urinary analgesics, nonsteroidal anti-inflammatory drugs, non-opioid medications, and opioid analgesia. A comprehensive program may be needed to adequately manage pain.[1]

Patient enrollment in research trials should be considered at any point in the treatment process.[1,2] The Multidisciplinary Approach to the Study of Chronic Pelvic Pain Research Network is one resource (https://www.niddk.nih.gov/news/archive/2016/multidisciplinary-approach-study-chronic-pelvic-pain).

SELF-MANAGEMENT STRATEGIES

For self-management strategies recommended for all patients, see **Box 2**.

Dietary Modification

The reasons certain foods and beverages trigger symptoms in BPS is poorly understood, but 90% of patients report that their symptoms do change with their diet.[19–21] Because an elimination diet is safe and relatively inexpensive, all patients should be advised to eliminate common triggers and monitor their symptoms with reintroduction to identify their specific triggers (**Box 3**). A list of common trigger foods and helpful dietary information for patients can be found on the IC Association Web site (www.ichelp.org).

Stress Reduction

Because of the affect that BPS can have on a patient's lifestyle, most patients will benefit from referral to psychological services to learn with strategies to manage the stress associated with the pain, such as relaxation exercises and reframing of symptoms.[1,22] For the subset of patients who have a predominant psychosomatic cause, psychological services will be even more important.[23]

Fluid Management

Patients should also be counseled to drink enough water to adequately flush out the bladder on a regular basis.[21,24] This need must be weighed against the patient's desire to avoid urinary frequency. Adequate hydration can also help prevent constipation, which can exacerbate symptoms in BPS.

Bladder Retraining

Bladder retraining helps treat urinary frequency by increasing the time between voids.[22,24] Because patients with BPS often void to relieve discomfort, bladder retraining should be delayed until pain is improved.[25,26]

Box 2
Self-management strategies recommended for all patients

- Dietary modification (avoiding trigger foods)
- Stress reduction
- Fluid management
- Bladder retraining

Box 3
Common diet triggers in BPS

- Acidic foods
  - Citrus fruits and juices
  - Tomatoes
  - Vinegar
  - Pickled foods
  - Fermented foods (eg, sauerkraut)
- Spicy foods
- Vitamin C
- Artificial sweeteners
- Coffee (both caffeinated and decaffeinated)
- Tea
- Carbonated beverages
- Alcohol

NON-PHARMACOLOGIC STRATEGIES

Pelvic Floor Physical Therapy and Myofascial Release

Pelvic floor physical therapy is often very effective and should be recommended for most patients. Physical therapy aims to treat hypertonic pelvic floor muscles. Guidelines advocate avoidance of methods that strengthen pelvic floor muscles, as this can increase pelvic floor tightness.[1,2] One study showed a 94% decrease in symptomatology with a manual physical therapy and myofascial release treatment program.[27]

Acupuncture

One study reported a greater than 50% reduction of pelvic pain in 11 of 14 patients treated with up to 8 weeks of acupuncture therapy twice a week.[18] Another study reported a 73% reduction in pain after acupuncture treatment compared with only a 47% pain reduction with sham acupuncture in men with chronic pelvic pain.[28] Most studies remain poor quality or underpowered and more research is needed. However, because acupuncture is safe and relatively inexpensive, it is recommended as an option.[1,2,24]

Neurostimulation

There is poor quality evidence and limited support for transcutaneous nerve stimulation units. A transcutaneous nerve stimulation unit stimulates peripheral sensory nerves and prevents nerve impulses contributing to chronic pain from reaching the brain. It has the advantage of being available in an outpatient setting, and does not require any procedures to place. Some studies have shown improvement with continuous, daily use, but treatments may take months to show significant effect.[29]

PHARMACOLOGIC STRATEGIES

Oral Therapies

Oral medications are second-line therapies for treatment of BPS[1,2,12] that should be added to conservative treatments when needed. **Table 2** summarizes the options.

Pentosan polysulfate (PPS) is the only oral medication that is U.S. Food and Drug Administration (FDA) approved for treatment of BPS.[30] A recent placebo-controlled

Table 2
Oral therapies

Oral Therapy	Dose	Associated Symptom Phenotypes	Notes
Amitriptyline	25–75 mg orally qHS	Bladder-specific, Hunner's lesions absent	Initiate at 10 mg qHS and titrate up weekly[29]
Cimetidine	400 mg orally twice a day	Bladder-specific, Hunner's lesions absent Neurologic/Systemic	
Hydroxyzine	10–50 mg orally qHS	Bladder-specific, Hunner's lesions absent Neurologic/Systemic	
Gabapentin	300–2100 mg orally divided 3 times a day	Neurologic/Systemic	
Pentosane polysulfate (PPS)	100 mg orally 3 times a day	Bladder-specific, Hunner's lesions absent	Only medication FDA approved for BPS Check LFTs 6 mo after starting treatment
Cyclosporine A	2–3 mg/kg divided twice a day	Bladder-specific, Hunner's lesions present	Fifth-line treatment, for severe/refractory cases Due to potential for adverse events, use limited to experienced clinicians
Phenazopyridine (pyridium)	200 mg orally 3 times a day	Acute flares	Not to be used for more than 2 d

Abbreviations: BPS, bladder pain syndrome; FDA, U.S. food and drug administration; LFTs, liver function tests; qHS, at bedtime.

trial of 368 patients failed to show any statistically significant difference between oral PPS and placebo.[31] In light of this evidence and the adverse effect profile, the Royal College of Obstetricians & Gynaecologists (RCOG) and the British Society of Urogynaecology (BSUG) no longer recommend PPS for treatment of BPS.[32] The American Urological Association (AUA) judged that the balance between benefits and risks/burdens was relatively equal and similar to other oral treatments and therefore designated it as an option, noting lower efficacy in patients with Hunner's lesions.[1]

In a randomized control trial, amitriptyline (25 mg daily titrated over several weeks to 100 mg if tolerated) was shown to be superior to placebo (63% of treatment group clinically improved compared with 4% of placebo group at 4 months).[33] The adverse effect profile, including dry mouth, constipation, sedation, weight gain, blurred vision, and nausea often limits compliance, with observational studies reporting up to 79% adverse reaction rate.[1,32,34]

Several observational studies have suggested that hydroxyzine and cimetidine are effective. Cimetidine was shown to achieve statistically significant improvement in bladder symptom scores in one randomized control trial.[35] Treatment with hydroxyzine did not show statistically significant response rate versus placebo in another randomized control trial.[36] For this reason, RCOG/BSUG does not recommend hydroxyzine, but it is still recommended by the AUA and the Canadian Urological Association.

Cyclosporine A is only recommended for refractory cases after patients have failed all other therapies. Observational studies and one randomized control trial have shown sustained efficacy, especially in those patients with Hunner's lesions identified on cystoscopy. However, it has the potential for serious adverse events, including nephrotoxicity and immunosuppression, and requires close patient monitoring with serum drug concentrations.[1,2,12,32]

Intravesicular Therapies

Intravesicular therapies, which require referral to a urologist or urogynecologist, are the direct introduction of pharmacologic treatment into the bladder via a catheter.[1,2] The treatments should be considered to confirm the diagnosis and rule out other causes of chronic pain, as well as in those patients with severe symptoms who do not improve with less invasive treatments.[1,2,12] The most common intravesicular therapies are dimethyl sulfoxide, lidocaine, and heparin. Low-pressure, short-term hydrodistension has also been used. These therapies are often used individually or used together mixed in a "cocktail" that is instilled into the bladder. Most have limited data on effectiveness and provide relief for only a short period of time.[37] Monthly maintenance therapy for those who respond is recommended.[1,2] Dimethyl sulfoxide (the only FDA-approved intravesicular treatment) is typically instilled weekly for 6 weeks. The procedure is invasive and the most common side effect is pain.[37,38]

Discouraged Treatments

Long-term oral antibiotics and systemic steroids are not recommended.[1,2]

REFRACTIVE DISEASE

BPS requires a multidisciplinary approach to care, which focuses on maximizing function. A diagnosis of BPS should not preclude evaluation for other diagnoses if new symptoms develop.[23] The BPS diagnosis should be reconsidered if no improvement occurs after multiple treatment approaches and ineffective treatments should be discontinued after a clinically meaningful interval has elapsed.[1] Chronic inflammatory diseases, including BPS, are risk factors for bladder cancer; no screening guidelines exist at this time, but new hematuria should prompt consideration of cystoscopy.[39] In addition, patients with this inflammatory disease may be at risk for a wide range of other medical conditions.[40,41] Surgical intervention should be reserved only for severe, refractory cases.[1,2]

SUMMARY

BPS is one of several causes of chronic pelvic pain, with patients having lower urinary symptoms in addition to bladder discomfort. Like all chronic pain conditions, treatment should focus on maximizing function with a combination of lifestyle changes and pharmacotherapy. For BPS, dietary modifications and physical therapy are especially helpful. Amitriptyline, gabapentin, cimetidine, and hydroxyzine are reasonable options for patients not controlled with non-pharmacological measures. Refractive and severe cases should be referred to urology for consideration of intravesicular treatments.

REFERENCES

1. Hanno PM, Burks DA, Clemens JQ, et al. AUA guideline for the diagnosis and treatment of interstitial cystitis/bladder pain syndrome. J Urol 2014;185(6): 2162–70.

2. Cox A, Golda N, Nadeau G, et al. CUA guideline: diagnosis and treatment of interstitial cystitis/bladder pain syndrome. Can Urol Assoc J 2016;10(5–6):E136.
3. Suskind AM, Berry SH, Ewing BA, et al. The prevalence and overlap of interstitial cystitis/bladder pain syndrome and chronic prostatitis/chronic pelvic pain syndrome in men; results of the RAND Interstitial Cystitis Epidemiology (RICE) Male Study. J Urol 2013;189(1):141–5.
4. Professionals S-O. Chronic pelvic pain. Uroweb. Available at: https://uroweb.org/guideline/chronic-pelvic-pain/. Accessed June 11, 2018.
5. McLennan MT. Interstitial cystitis: epidemiology, pathophysiology, and clinical presentation. Obstet Gynecol Clin North Am 2014;41(3):385–95.
6. Clemens JQ, Joyce GF, Wise M, et al. Interstitial cystitis and painful bladder syndrome. Washington, DC: US Department of Health and Human Services, Public Health, National Institutes of Health, National Institute of Diabetes and Digestive and Kidney Diseases; 2007. p. 125–54.
7. Berry SH, Elliott MN, Suttorp M, et al. Prevalence of symptoms of bladder pain syndrome/interstitial cystitis among adult females in the United States. J Urol 2011;186(2):540–4.
8. Jhang J-F, Kuo H-C. Pathomechanism of interstitial cystitis/bladder pain syndrome and mapping the heterogeneity of disease. Int Neurourol J 2016; 20(Suppl 2):S95–104.
9. Sant GR. Etiology, pathogenesis, and diagnosis of interstitial cystitis. Rev Urol 2002;4(Suppl 1):S9–15.
10. Grover S, Srivastava A, Lee R, et al. Role of inflammation in bladder function and interstitial cystitis. Ther Adv Urol 2011;3(1):19–33.
11. van de Merwe JP, Nordling J, Bouchelouche P, et al. Diagnostic criteria, classification, and nomenclature for painful bladder syndrome/interstitial cystitis: an ESSIC proposal. Eur Urol 2008;53(1):60–7.
12. Malde S, Palmisani S, Al-Kaisy A, et al. Guideline of guidelines: bladder pain syndrome. BJU Int 2018. https://doi.org/10.1111/bju.14399.
13. Morgan TM, Clark PE. Bladder cancer. Curr Opin Oncol 2010;22(3):242–9.
14. Bladder cancer risk factors. Available at: https://www.cancer.org/cancer/bladder-cancer/causes-risks-prevention/risk-factors.html. Accessed July 26, 2018.
15. Cox A. Management of interstitial cystitis/bladder pain syndrome. Can Urol Assoc J 2018;12(6 Suppl 3):S157–60.
16. Beckett MK, Elliott MN, Clemens JQ, et al. Consequences of interstitial cystitis/bladder pain symptoms on women's work participation and income: results from a national household sample. J Urol 2014;191(1):83–8.
17. Bosch PC. Examination of the significant placebo effect in the treatment of interstitial cystitis/bladder pain syndrome. Urology 2014;84(2):321–6.
18. Rapkin AJ, Kames LD. The pain management approach to chronic pelvic pain. J Reprod Med 1987;32(5):323–7.
19. Friedlander JI, Shorter B, Moldwin RM. Diet and its role in interstitial cystitis/bladder pain syndrome (IC/BPS) and comorbid conditions: DIET AND ITS ROLE IN IC/BPS AND COMORBID CONDITIONS. BJU Int 2012;109(11):1584–91.
20. Bassaly R, Downes K, Hart S. Dietary consumption triggers in interstitial cystitis/bladder pain syndrome patients. Female Pelvic Med Reconstr Surg 2011;17(1):36–9.
21. Gordon B, Shorter B, Sarcona A, et al. Nutritional considerations for patients with interstitial cystitis/bladder pain syndrome. J Acad Nutr Diet 2015;115(9):1372–9.

22. Verghese TS, Riordain RN, Champaneria R, et al. Complementary therapies for bladder pain syndrome: a systematic review. Int Urogynecol J 2016;27:1127–36.
23. Warren JW. Bladder pain syndrome/interstitial cystitis as a functional somatic syndrome. J Psychosom Res 2014;77(6):510–5.
24. Whitmore KE. Complementary and alternative therapies as treatment approaches for interstitial cystitis. Rev Urol 2002;4(Suppl 1):S28–35.
25. Parsons CL, Koprowski PF. Interstitial cystitis: successful management by increasing urinary voiding intervals. Urology 1991;37(3):207–12.
26. Chaiken DC, Blaivas JG, Blaivas ST. Behavioral therapy for the treatment of refractory interstitial cystitis. J Urol 1993;149(6):1445–8.
27. Lukban J, Whitmore K, Kellogg-Spadt S, et al. The effect of manual physical therapy in patients diagnosed with interstitial cystitis, high-tone pelvic floor dysfunction, and sacroiliac dysfunction. Urology 2001;57(6 Suppl 1):121–2.
28. Lee S-H, Lee B-C. Use of acupuncture as a treatment method for chronic prostatitis/chronic pelvic pain syndromes. Curr Urol Rep 2011;12(4):288–96.
29. Fall M, Carlsson C-A, Erlandson B-E. Electrical stimulation in interstitial cystitis. J Urol 1980;123(2):192–5.
30. Payne CK, Joyce GF, Wise M, et al, Urologic diseases in America Project. Interstitial cystitis and painful bladder syndrome. J Urol 2007;177(6):2042–9.
31. Nickel JC, Herschorn S, Whitmore KE, et al. Pentosan polysulfate sodium for treatment of interstitial cystitis/bladder pain syndrome: insights from a randomized, double-blind, placebo controlled study. J Urol 2015;193(3):857–62.
32. Management of bladder pain syndrome: green-top guideline no. 70. BJOG 2017; 124(2):e46–72.
33. van Ophoven A, Pokupic S, Heinecke A, et al. A prospective, randomized, placebo controlled, double-blind study of amitriptyline for the treatment of interstitial cystitis. J Urol 2004;172(2):533–6.
34. van Ophoven A, Hertle L. Long-term results of amitriptyline treatment for interstitial cystitis. J Urol 2005;174(5):1837–40.
35. Thilagarajah R, Witherow RO, Walker MM. Oral cimetidine gives effective symptom relief in painful bladder disease: a prospective, randomized, double-blind placebo-controlled trial. BJU Int 2001;87(3):207–12.
36. Sant GR, Propert KJ, Hanno PM, et al. A pilot clinical trial of oral pentosan polysulfate and oral hydroxyzine in patients with interstitial cystitis. J Urol 2003;170(3): 810–5.
37. Colaco MA, Evans RJ. Current recommendations for bladder instillation therapy in the treatment of interstitial cystitis/bladder pain syndrome. Curr Urol Rep 2013;14(5):442–7.
38. Dyer AJ, Twiss CO. Painful bladder syndrome: an update and review of current management strategies. Curr Urol Rep 2014;15(2):384.
39. Keller J, Chiou H-Y, Lin H-C. Increased risk of bladder cancer following diagnosis with bladder pain syndrome/interstitial cystitis. Neurourol Urodyn 2013;32(1): 58–62.
40. Chen H-M, Lin C-C, Kang C-S, et al. Bladder pain syndrome/interstitial cystitis increase the risk of coronary heart disease. Neurourol Urodyn 2014;33(5):511–5.
41. Chung S-D, Xirasagar S, Lin C-C, et al. Increased risk of ischemic stroke among women with bladder pain syndrome/interstitial cystitis: a cohort study from Taiwan. Neurourol Urodyn 2015;34(1):44–9.

Benign Prostatic Hyperplasia

Robert C. Langan, MD[a,b,*]

KEYWORDS

- Benign prostatic hyperplasia • Lower urinary tract symptoms
- Alpha-adrenergic blockers • 5-alpha reductase inhibitors
- Transurethral resection of the prostate

KEY POINTS

- Lower urinary tract symptoms (LUTS), which may be obstructive, irritative, or both, are most commonly the result of benign prostatic hyperplasia (BPH) in aging men.
- The American Urologic Association Symptom Index is a validated scoring system that allows physicians to assess the severity of LUTS, suggest initial treatment, and monitor the response to treatment.
- Watchful waiting is a reasonable approach to men with mild LUTS due to BPH.
- Effective pharmacotherapy for BPH includes both alpha-adrenergic blockers and 5-alpha reductase inhibitors.
- Surgical procedures, including less invasive modalities, are generally indicated for failure of medical therapy, refractory urinary retention, recurrent urinary tract infection, persistent hematuria, bladder stones, or renal insufficiency.

OVERVIEW

Benign prostatic hyperplasia (BPH) is the most common benign neoplasm of aging men and is present in approximately 8% of men in the fourth decade of life but up to 90% of men in the ninth decade.[1] BPH refers to the change in the size of the prostate and not the potential symptoms that it may cause, which are usually referred to as lower urinary tract symptoms (LUTS). LUTS may be primarily irritative, obstructive, or mixed. Men with BPH may be asymptomatic, respond to lifestyle changes, or require medical or surgical therapy; symptoms are more common as men age. Once primarily treated by urologists, guidelines now emphasize a primary care approach.[2,3]

Disclosure Statement: The author has nothing to disclose.

[a] St. Luke's Family Medicine Residency, Sacred Heart Campus, 450 Chew Street, Suite 101, Allentown, PA 18102, USA; [b] Department of Family and Community Medicine, Temple University School of Medicine, Philadelphia, PA, USA
* 450 Chew Street, Suite 101, Allentown, PA 18102.
E-mail address: Robert.Langan@sluhn.org

Prim Care Clin Office Pract 46 (2019) 223–232
https://doi.org/10.1016/j.pop.2019.02.003

The prostate is an almond-shaped gland located at the junction of the urinary bladder and the urethra in men. Its name derives from the Greek expression for "one who stands before," referring to its anatomic location. It secretes a milky, alkaline fluid that constitutes approximately 30% of the volume of semen. It is covered by a capsule of connective tissue that contains smooth muscle fibers and elastic tissue. Within the capsule, 3 zones are identified: (1) the transition zone, located closest to the urethra; (2) the central zone, where the common duct from the prostate and seminal vesicles is found; and (3) the large peripheral zone. The normal volume of the prostate gland is approximately 20 to 30 g.

PATHOPHYSIOLOGY AND RISK FACTORS

The pathophysiology of BPH is incompletely understood.[4] Histologically, hyperplasia of glandular elements in the periurethral zone and stromal elements in the transition zone are responsible for the symptoms reported by men and are dependent on the bioavailability of both testosterone and dihydrotestosterone (DHT).[5] There is no clear correlation between prostate size on physical examination and symptom severity.[6] So-called static symptoms are due to simple anatomic obstruction, whereas dynamic symptoms are mediated through a number of receptors (alpha-adrenergic,[7] muscarinic,[8] and phosphodiesterase-5 [PDE-5]).[9] These receptors are the target for pharmacotherapy.

In addition to increasing age, risk factors for the development of BPH include African American race,[10] obesity,[11] type 2 diabetes mellitus,[12] high levels of alcohol consumption,[13] and physical inactivity.[14]

PRESENTATION AND ASSESSMENT

Men with symptomatic BPH may present with obstructive symptoms, irritative symptoms, or a combination of both (**Table 1**). The American Urologic Association Symptom Index (AUASI)[15] is a validated, self-administered, quantitative measure of the severity of LUTS due to BPH (**Box 1**). The AUASI score ranges from 0 (no symptoms) to 35 (severe symptoms). In addition to diagnosis of BPH, the AUASI can aid in selecting initial therapy (see Pharmacologic and Surgical Treatment sections) and monitoring the response to therapy; a 3-point change on the AUASI scale is considered significant.[16] In addition to the 7 symptom questions, an eighth question is often added to assess quality of life due to BPH: If you were to spend the rest of your life with your urinary condition just the way it is now, how would you feel about this? Scores for this question range from 0 (delighted) to 6 (terrible).[17] This 8-question symptom index is called the International Prostate Symptom Score.

A number of medications may cause LUTS.[18] Excessive alcohol, caffeine, or diuretic use may result in diuresis. Anticholinergic medications, such as dicyclomine, impair

Table 1
Lower urinary tract symptoms of benign prostatic hyperplasia

Obstructive Symptoms	Irritative Symptoms
1. Sensation of incomplete bladder emptying	1. Dysuria
2. Straining to void	2. Nocturia
3. Urinary hesitancy	3. Urinary frequency
4. Weak urinary stream	4. Urinary urgency

Data from Sarma AV, Wei JT. Benign prostatic hyperplasia and lower urinary tract symptoms. N Engl J Med 2012;367(3):248–57.

Box 1
American Urologic Association symptom index

In the past month, how often have you experienced the following symptoms?[a]
1. Sensation of not completely emptying your bladder
2. Need to urinate less than 2 hours after urinating
3. Stopped and started again while urinating
4. Found it difficult to postpone urination
5. Had a weak urinary stream
6. Had to push or strain to begin urinating
7. How many times do you get up at night to urinate?[b]

[a] Scoring for questions 1 to 6: 0: Not at all; 1: Less than 20% of the time; 2: Less than 50% of the time; 3: 50% of the time; 4: More than 50% of the time; 5: All of the time.
[b] Scoring for question 7: Each time is worth 1 point (maximum of 5 points)
Total score is the sum of the scores for questions 1 to 7 (minimum 0, maximum 35)
Adapted from Barry MJ, Fowler FJ Jr, O'Leary MP, et al. The American Urological Association symptom index for benign prostatic hyperplasia. J Urol 1992;148:1555; with permission.

contractility of the smooth muscle of the urinary tract and may cause obstructive symptoms. First-generation antihistamines, including diphenhydramine, increase outlet obstruction. Other medications that may produce LUTS are alpha-agonists, beta-blockers, and calcium channel blockers. If feasible, potentially offending medications should be stopped to see if symptoms improve.

On physical examination, a digital rectal examination (DRE) should be done to assess sphincter tone, prostate size, and the presence of prostate nodules or masses. If a nodule or mass is noted, urology consultation for potential biopsy is recommended. DRE tends to underestimate the prostate volume.[19] A focused neurologic examination should be done to assess for neurologic diseases that might produce LUTS.

A limited laboratory assessment should be done in men with suspected BPH. A urinalysis is recommended to exclude infection, which can produce LUTS, and hematuria, which is not typically seen in BPH and should prompt further evaluation.[20] If infection is detected, it should be treated before initiating therapy specific for BPH. Prostate-specific antigen (PSA) testing can be considered for men who are have at least a 10-year life expectancy and desire screening, after an appropriate discussion of its risks and limited benefits.[20] PSA may be used to estimate the size of the prostate.[21] Of note, PSA is not useful for differentiating BPH from prostate cancer. If urinary obstruction is suspected, renal function should be assessed with a serum blood urea nitrogen and creatinine, and ultrasound of the bladder to measure residual volume should be done.[22] Otherwise, imaging tests and urodynamics are generally not indicated for men with suspected BPH.

NONPHARMACOLOGIC TREATMENT

In men with mild LUTS symptoms from BPH (usually defined as an AUASI score of 0–7), medical or surgical treatment is not required. In the Medical Therapy of Prostatic Symptoms Study,[23] fewer than 5% of men with mild symptoms who did not receive treatment had a progression of their symptoms as defined by a 4-point or greater increase in their AUASI score. No cases of acute kidney injury due to obstructive uropathy occurred. Men who choose nonpharmacologic treatment (**Box 2**) should be reassessed annually with the AUASI.

Box 2
Nonpharmacologic management of lower urinary tract symptoms

1. Moderate use of alcohol
2. Moderate use of caffeine
3. Avoid medications that may produce lower urinary tract symptoms
4. Limit salt intake
5. Maintain a time voiding schedule
6. Limit fluid intake 1 to 2 hours before sleep

Data from McVary KT, Roehrborn CG, Avins AL, et al. Update on AUA guideline on the management of benign prostatic hyperplasia. J Urol 2011;185(5):1793–803.

PHARMACOLOGIC TREATMENT

Men with moderate to severe LUTS from BPH (AUASI score of 8 or higher) or mild LUTS that are deemed bothersome by the patient may be offered pharmacologic treatment. The 2 major classes of medications for BPH are alpha-adrenergic blockers and 5-alpha reductase inhibitors. The PDE-5 inhibitor tadalafil is also approved by the Food and Drug Administration (FDA) for the treatment of BPH. Many men also are interested in the use of alternative therapy to treat LUTS.

ALPHA-ADRENERGIC BLOCKERS

The smooth muscle of the prostate and bladder neck is under the control of alpha-adrenergic nerves. Stimulation of these sympathetic nerve fibers is associated with contraction of the smooth muscle and an increase in dynamic urinary obstruction.[7] The alpha-adrenergic blockers ("alpha blockers") were originally developed as antihypertensive agents, but fell out of favor after the alpha-blocker doxazosin was found to have higher rates of stroke and combined cardiovascular events when compared with a thiazide diuretic in the ALLHAT trial.[24] However, their utility at blocking the sympathetic fibers in the prostate and bladder and improving LUTS has led to their widespread use for this indication.

Alpha blockers are further subdivided based on their selectivity for alpha-adrenergic receptors located in the urinary tract. There does not seem to be a significant difference in the efficacy of these agents.[25,26] On average, alpha blockers will reduce an AUASI score by 4 to 6 points.[4] Symptom relief typically occurs within 1 week after starting therapy, but may take as long as 4 weeks to achieve.

Nonselective alpha blockers carry the highest risk of orthostatic hypotension,[27] and should be started at a low dose and titrated up over the period of a few weeks. They are also associated with an increased risk of falls and fractures.[28] In general, alpha blockers should not be combined with PDE-5 inhibitors due to the risk of hypotension.[29] In 2005, there were reports of progressive intraoperative miosis, billowing and flaccid iris, and prolapse of the iris toward the incision site in men who had recently started alpha blockers and were undergoing cataract surgery.[30] This condition was later termed intraoperative floppy iris syndrome, and the risk appears to be highest in men taking tamsulosin. It is recommended that men who are planning on cataract surgery in the next few weeks to months should not be started on an alpha-blocker.[31] However, it is unclear if men who have been taking alpha blockers should stop it before surgery or how long after surgery alpha blockers may be safely started.

Alpha blockers are listed in **Table 2**.

Table 2
Alpha-adrenergic blockers

Type	Drug	Dose	Side Effects
Nonselective	Doxazosin Terazosin	1 mg daily; titrate to maximum dose of 8 mg daily 1 mg daily; titrate to maximum dose of 20 mg daily	• Rhinitis • Headache • Orthostatic hypotension (avoid use of phosphodiesterase-5 inhibitors and titrate dose slowly)
Selective	Alfuzosin Silodosin Tamsulosin	10 mg daily 8 mg daily 0.4 mg daily; titrate to maximum of 0.8 mg daily	• Retrograde ejaculation • Rhinitis • Intraoperative floppy iris syndrome (tamsulosin)

Data from Sarma AV, Wei JT. Benign prostatic hyperplasia and lower urinary tract symptoms. N Engl J Med 2012;367(3):248–57.

5-ALPHA REDUCTASE INHIBITORS

Prostatic tissue is stimulated by both testosterone and its metabolite DHT, which is produced through the action of the enzyme 5-alpha reductase. Blocking the action of 5-alpha reductase has the benefit of reducing the stimulation of prostatic tissue through reduction of levels of DHT while preserving the androgen effects of testosterone. The available 5-alpha reductase inhibitors, finasteride and dutasteride, reduce prostate size by as much as 25% and reduce the AUASI score by 4 to 5 points in men with larger prostates, although over a much longer period than is seen with alpha-adrenergic blockers (typically 2–6 months) (**Table 3**).[32] Unlike alpha-adrenergic blockers, 5-alpha reductase inhibitors are associated with a reduced risk of acute urinary retention (number needed to treat of 26) and surgical intervention (number needed to treat of 18) after 4 years.[33] Although dutasteride inhibits both subsets of 5-alpha reductase and finasteride inhibits only one, their efficacy appears to be similar.[34] The 5-alpha reductase inhibitors should be used only in men with large prostates as determined by DRE, ultrasound, or the use of a surrogate marker, such as PSA.

Side effects of 5-alpha reductase inhibitors include decreased libido, erectile dysfunction, decreased ejaculation, and gynecomastia.[32] Because prostate cancer is also stimulated by DHT, trials were undertaken to assess if these medications could be used to reduce the risk of developing neoplasms of the prostate. Use of either agent was associated with a 6% absolute risk reduction in the development of prostate cancer but also an increased risk of developing a moderate-risk to high-risk prostate cancer for unknown reasons.[35–37] Consequently, 5-alpha reductase inhibitors are not recommended as chemoprophylaxis against the development of prostate cancer. Because PSA levels decrease by approximately 50% after 6 months of therapy, any significant increase in PSA should prompt urologic evaluation.[4]

COMBINATION ALPHA-ADRENERGIC BLOCKERS/5-ALPHA REDUCTASE INHIBITORS

A number of trials have explored the use of combinations of alpha-adrenergic blockers and 5-alpha reductase inhibitors in the treatment of LUTS.[23,38] Combinations including doxazosin with finasteride and tamsulosin with dutasteride demonstrated superior improvement in AUASI scores when compared with each component alone. The American Urologic Association lists combination therapy as an option, stating

Table 3
5-alpha reductase inhibitors

Drug	Enzyme Inhibited	Dose	Side Effects
Finasteride	5-alpha reductase, type 2	5 mg daily	• Abnormal ejaculation
Dutasteride	5-alpha reductase, types 1 and 2	0.5 mg daily	• Decreased prostate-specific antigen level
			• Erectile dysfunction
			• Gynecomastia
			• Increased risk of high-grade prostate cancer

Data from Sarma AV, Wei JT. Benign prostatic hyperplasia and lower urinary tract symptoms. N Engl J Med 2012;367(3):248–57.

that, "The combination of an alpha-blocker and a 5α-reductase inhibitor (combination therapy) is an appropriate and effective treatment for patients with LUTS associated with demonstrable prostatic enlargement based on volume measurement, PSA level as a proxy for volume, and/or enlargement on DRE."[20] Fixed-dose combination therapy is more expensive than the individual components and combination therapy is associated with more side effects. Currently, the only fixed-dose product available in the United States is dutasteride 0.5 mg/tamsulosin 0.4 mg.

PHOSPHODIESTERASE-5 INHIBITORS

As previously mentioned, PDE-5 is present throughout prostatic tissue, the bladder detrusor muscle, and vascular smooth muscle that is associated with the urinary tract.[9] The PDE-5 inhibitors, which were initially approved by the FDA for the treatment of erectile dysfunction, may also improve LUTS. When PDE-5 is inhibited, the resulting increase in cyclic AMP and cyclic guanosine monophosphate relaxes smooth muscle. Of the available PDE-5 inhibitors, only tadalafil has been approved for the treatment of LUTS from BPH. In a 12-week trial, daily tadalafil improved the AUASI by 3.8 points.[39] Side effects include headache, indigestion, back pain, flushing, and nasal congestion. Combining tadalafil with an alpha-adrenergic blocker or nitrate can cause symptomatic hypotension.[29]

COMPLEMENTARY MEDICATIONS

A number of herbal supplements have been tried for the treatment of LUTS. Perhaps the most extensively studied has been saw palmetto (*Serenoa repens*), but a 2012 Cochrane review concluded that it did not improve urinary flow or prostate size.[40] There is insufficient evidence to support the use of other supplements, such as African plum bark, purple cone flower roots, stinging nettle, South African star grass, rye pollen extract, or pumpkin seeds.[20]

SURGICAL THERAPIES

Several procedures are available for the treatment of symptomatic BPH. General indications for surgical treatment are listed in **Box 3**. The most commonly performed surgical procedure is transurethral resection of the prostate (TURP), which is considered the gold standard. Men should be screened for urinary tract infection as part of a preoperative evaluation; if present, it should be treated before surgery. Potential complications include retrograde ejaculation, erectile dysfunction, hematuria, urethral

Box 3
Indications for surgical treatment of benign prostatic hypertrophy

1. Failure of medical therapy
2. Refractory urinary retention
3. Recurrent urinary tract infection
4. Persistent hematuria
5. Bladder stones
6. Renal insufficiency

Data from McVary KT, Roehrborn CG, Avins AL, et al. Update on AUA guideline on the management of benign prostatic hyperplasia. J Urol 2011;185(5):1793–803.

stricture, and urinary tract infection. Approximately 5% to 10% of men who undergo TURP will require a repeat procedure with 10 years.[20]

A number of less invasive procedures have been developed for the treatment of BPH. In general, these procedures are associated with less morbidity than TURP but are also associated with a higher risk of need for retreatment. Healthy men with low surgical risk are appropriate for TURP, whereas men with higher surgical risk or who cannot tolerate general anesthesia may require less invasive surgical treatment. Examples of these procedures include photoselective vaporization of the prostate, transurethral incision of the prostate, transurethral laser prostatectomy, and transurethral microwave prostate.

Prostatic urethral lift is a noninvasive procedure in which a permanent implant is placed via cystoscopy that relieves the obstruction from BPH. Studies have shown that it produces an improvement in AUASI of up to 11 points in as early as 3 months,[41] and these improvements have been shown to persist after 5 years.[42] Unlike TURP, prostatic urethral lift is not associated with side effects such as erectile dysfunction or retrograde ejaculation.[43] Patients should have large (greater than 100 g) prostates that can be compressed with a rigid cystoscope.

SUMMARY

In summary, BPH is a common condition in aging men that is frequently associated with troublesome LUTS. The AUASI is a validated, self-administered tool that can be used to diagnose LUTS, guide initial treatment, and assess response to treatment. Watchful waiting is a reasonable option for men with mild symptoms. The mainstay of pharmacologic treatment is alpha-adrenergic blockers and 5-alpha reductase inhibitors. There is no evidence to support the use of herbal supplements in the treatment of LUTS. Surgical therapy is effective and is indicated for men with complications from BPH or who fail medical therapy.

REFERENCES

1. McVary KT. BPH: epidemiology and comorbidities. Am J Manag Care 2006;12(5 suppl):S122–8.
2. Kapoor A. Benign prostatic hyperplasia (BPH) management in the primary care setting. Can J Urol 2012;19(Suppl 1):10–7.
3. Jones C, Hill J, Chapple C, on behalf of the Guideline Development Group. Management of lower urinary tract symptoms in men: summary of the NICE guidelines. BMJ 2010;340:c2354.

4. Sarma AV, Wei JT. Benign prostatic hyperplasia and lower urinary tract symptoms. N Engl J Med 2012;367(3):248–57.
5. Bartsch G, Rittmaster RS, Klocker H. Dihydrotestosterone and the concept of 5-alpha-reductase inhibition in human benign prostatic hyperplasia. Eur Urol 2000;37:367–80.
6. Simon RM, Howard LE, Moreira DM, et al. Does prostate size predict the development of incident lower urinary tract symptoms in men with mild to no current symptoms? Results from the REDUCE trial. Eur Urol 2016;69:885–91.
7. Schwinn DA, Roehrborn CG. α1-Adrenoceptor subtypes and lower urinary tract symptoms. Int J Urol 2008;15:193–9.
8. Andersson KE. Antimuscarinics for the treatment of overactive bladder. Lancet Neurol 2004;3:46–53.
9. Andersson KE, de Groat WC, McVary KT, et al. Tadalafil for the treatment of lower urinary tract symptoms secondary to benign prostatic hyperplasia: pathophysiology and mechanism(s) of action. Neurourol Urodyn 2011;30:292–301.
10. Kristal AR, Arnold KB, Schenk JM, et al. Race/ethnicity, obesity, health related behaviors and the risk of symptomatic benign prostatic hyperplasia: results from the prostate cancer prevention trial. J Urol 2007;177:1395–400.
11. Giovannucci E, Rimm EB, Chute CG, et al. Obesity and benign prostatic hyperplasia. Am J Epidemiol 1994;140:989–1002.
12. Sarma AV, St Sauver JL, Hollingsworth JM, et al. Diabetes treatment and progression of benign prostatic hyperplasia in community-dwelling black and white men. Urology 2012;79:102–8.
13. Parsons JK, Im R. Alcohol consumption is associated with a decreased risk of benign prostatic hyperplasia. J Urol 2009;182:1463–8.
14. Platz EA, Kawachi I, Rimm EB, et al. Physical activity and benign prostatic hyperplasia. Arch Intern Med 1998;158:2349–56.
15. Barry MJ, Fowler FJ Jr, O'Leary MP, et al. The American Urological Association symptom index for benign prostatic hyperplasia. J Urol 1992;148:1549–57.
16. Barry MJ, Williford WO, Chang Y, et al. Benign prostatic hyperplasia specific health status measures in clinical research: how much change in the American Urological Association symptom index and the benign prostatic hyperplasia impact index is perceptible to patients? J Urol 1995;154:1770–4.
17. Wadie BS, Ibrahim EH, de la Rosette JJ, et al. The relationship of the International Prostate Symptom Score and objective parameters for diagnosing bladder outlet obstruction. Part I: when statistics fail. J Urol 2001;165(1):32–4.
18. Wuerstle MC, Van Den Eedern SK, Pook KT, et al. Contribution of common medications to lower urinary tract symptoms in men. Arch Intern Med 2011;171(18):1680–2.
19. Vuichoud C, Loughlin K. Benign prostatic hyperplasia: epidemiology, economics, and evaluation. Can J Urol 2015;22(Suppl 1):1–6.
20. McVary KT, Roehrborn CG, Avins AL, et al. Update on AUA guideline on the management of benign prostatic hyperplasia. J Urol 2011;185(5):1793–803.
21. Bohnen AM, Groeneveld FP, Bosch JL. Serum prostate-specific antigen as a predictor of prostate volume in the community: the Krimpen study. Eur Urol 2007;51(6):1645–52 [discussion: 1652–3].
22. McNeill SA, Hargreave TB, Geffriaud-Ricouard C, et al. Postvoid residual urine in patients with lower urinary tract symptoms suggestive of benign prostatic hyperplasia: pooled analysis of eleven controlled studies with alfuzosin. Urology 2001;57:459–65.

23. McConnell JD, Roehrborn CG, Bautista OM, et al. The long-term effect of doxazosin, finasteride, and combination therapy on the clinical progression of benign prostatic hyperplasia. N Engl J Med 2003;349(25):2387–98.
24. ALLHAT Officers, Coordinators for the ALLHAT Collaborative Research Group. Major cardiovascular events in hypertensive patients randomised to doxazosin vs chlorthalidone. The antihypertensive and lipid-lowering treatment to prevent heart attack trial (ALLHAT). JAMA 2000;283(15):1967–75.
25. Djavan B, Marberger M. A meta-analysis on the efficacy and tolerability of alpha1-adrenoceptor antagonists in patients with lower urinary tract symptoms suggestive of benign prostatic obstruction. Eur Urol 1999;36(1):1–13.
26. Jung J, Kim J, MacDonald R, et al. Silodosin for the treatment of lower urinary tract symptoms in men with benign prostatic hyperplasia. Cochrane Database Syst Rev 2017;(11):CD012615.
27. Chrischilles E, Rubenstein L, Chao J, et al. Initiation of nonselective alpha 1-antagonist therapy and occurrence of hypotension-related adverse events among men with benign prostatic hyperplasia: a retrospective cohort study. Clin Ther 2001;23:727–43.
28. Welk B, McArthur E, Fraser LA, et al. The risk of fall and fracture with the initiation of a prostate-selective α antagonist: a population based cohort study. BMJ 2015; 351:h5398.
29. Guillaume M, Lonsdale F, Darstein C, et al. Hemodynamic interaction between a daily dosed phosphodiesterase 5 inhibitor, tadalafil, and the alpha-adrenergic blockers, doxazosin and tamsulosin, in middle-aged healthy male subjects. J Clin Pharmacol 2007;47(10):1303–10.
30. Chang DF, Campbell JR. Intraoperative floppy iris syndrome associated with tamsulosin. J Cataract Refract Surg 2005;31:664–73.
31. Bell CM, Hatch WV, Fischer HD, et al. Association between tamsulosin and serious ophthalmic adverse events in older men following cataract surgery. JAMA 2009;301(19):1991–6.
32. Roehrborn CG. Male lower urinary tract symptoms (LUTS) and benign prostatic hyperplasia (BPH). Med Clin North Am 2011;95:87–100.
33. McConnell JD, Bruskewitz R, Walsh P, et al, for the Finasteride Long-Term Efficacy and Safety Study Group. The effect of finasteride on the risk of acute urinary retention and the need for surgical treatment among men with benign prostatic hyperplasia. N Engl J Med 1998;338(9):557–63.
34. Nickel JC, Gilling P, Tammela TL, et al. Comparison of dutasteride and finasteride for treating benign prostatic hyperplasia: the Enlarged Prostate International Comparator Study (EPICS). BJU Int 2011;108:388–94.
35. Thompson IM, Goodman PJ, Tangen CM, et al. The influence of finasteride on the development of prostate cancer. N Engl J Med 2003;349(3):215–24.
36. Thompson IM, Goodman PJ, Tangen CM, et al. Long-term survival of participants in the prostate cancer prevention trial. N Engl J Med 2013;369:603–10.
37. Walsh PC. Chemoprevention of prostate cancer. N Engl J Med 2010;362:1237.
38. Roehrborn CG, Siami P, Barkin J, et al. The effects of combination therapy with dutasteride and tamsulosin on clinical outcomes in men with symptomatic benign hyperplasia: 4-year results from the CombAT study. Eur Urol 2010;57:123–31.
39. McVary KT, Roehrborn CG, Kaminetsky JC, et al. Tadalafil relieves lower urinary tract symptoms secondary to benign prostatic hyperplasia. J Urol 2007;177: 1401–7.
40. Tacklind J, MacDonald R, Rutks I, et al. Serenoa repens for benign prostatic hyperplasia. Cochrane Database Syst Rev 2012;(12):CD001423.

41. Roehrborn CG, Gange SN, Shore ND, et al. The prostatic urethral life for treatment of urinary tract symptoms associated with prostate enlargement due to BPH: the LIFT Study. J Urol 2013;190(6):2161–7.
42. Roehrborn CG, Barkin J, Gange SN, et al. Five year results of the prospective randomized controlled prostatic urethral LIFT study. Can J Urol 2017;24(3):8802–13.
43. Sonksen J, Barber NJ, Speakman MJ, et al. Prospective, randomized, multinational study of prostatic urethral lift versus transurethral resection of the prostate: 12-month results from the BPH6 study. Eur Urol 2015;68(4):643–52.

Urinary Incontinence

Gretchen M. Irwin, MD, MBA

KEYWORDS

- Urinary incontinence • Stress incontinence • Urge incontinence
- Pelvic floor muscle training

KEY POINTS

- Many patients experience urinary incontinence but fail to report symptoms to a physician unless asked directly.
- Determining the type of urinary incontinence using history and physical examination is critical to effective treatment.
- The DIAPPERS mnemonic may help physicians recall reversible causes of urinary incontinence that should be ruled out in newly diagnosed individuals.
- Lifestyle modifications are helpful for urge, stress, and mixed incontinence.

INTRODUCTION

Urinary incontinence is a common, although often underreported, condition. Estimates suggest that approximately 20 million women and 6 million men in the United States experience urinary incontinence during their lives.[1] Furthermore, up to 77% of women in nursing homes may have urinary incontinence.[2] Despite such prevalence, only 25% of individuals affected by incontinence seek or receive treatment.[2] Nevertheless, urinary incontinence has significant impacts on quality of life and overall health for patients. Higher rates of depression and social isolation have been noted for patients with urinary incontinence.[3,4] Also, higher rates of hospitalization, urinary tract infection, pressure ulcers, and admission to long-term residential care as well as lower work productivity, general health, and quality of life are noted in populations with urinary incontinence compared with those without.[5–8] Although not often sought out, a variety of treatment options exist that can significantly improve symptoms. Lifestyle modifications, medications, and surgical options improve incontinence episode frequency and ultimately improve quality of life and general health for those individuals impacted.

Disclosure: The author has nothing to disclose.
Family Medicine Residency, Department of Family and Community Medicine, Wesley Medical Center, University of Kansas School of Medicine–Wichita, 1010 North Kansas, Wichita, KS 67214, USA
E-mail address: gdickson@kumc.edu

Prim Care Clin Office Pract 46 (2019) 233–242
https://doi.org/10.1016/j.pop.2019.02.004
primarycare.theclinics.com
0095-4543/19/

PATHOPHYSIOLOGY

Urinary incontinence can be defined simply as the loss of bladder control or unintentional voiding. Urinary incontinence can be classified as stress, urge, mixed, overflow, or functional. Defining the underlying cause of incontinence episodes is critical for appropriate treatment.

Stress incontinence develops when the urinary sphincter becomes weak and fails to function appropriately. Clinically, patients will note involuntary loss of urine with increased abdominal pressure, effort, or physical exertion.[9] Laughing, coughing, and exercise are common triggers of stress incontinence episodes. This type of incontinence is common in men after prostate surgery.[10] It is also common in women, as an estimated 50% of women under age 65 years with urinary incontinence have stress type.[11]

Urge incontinence results from overactivity of the detrusor muscle.[12] As the name suggests, a common patient complaint is involuntary loss of urine associated with feelings of extreme urgency to void with limited time to appropriately toilet.[9] The diagnosis of mixed incontinence should be given to patients who display features of both stress and urge type. Mixed incontinence is more common than urge type alone, as only 10% of women have isolated urge incontinence, whereas 30% have mixed type.[11] Although mixed incontinence is less common than stress type, studies have shown that women with mixed or urge incontinence may have lower quality-of-life scores than those with stress alone.[13]

Overflow incontinence results from obstruction or impaired detrusor contractility that leads to bladder distention, such as seen in men with benign prostatic hyperplasia leading to obstruction.[10,14]

Individuals may also suffer from functional incontinence, whereby cognitive or mobility impairment prevents an individual from appropriately toileting independently with no underlying bladder or neurologic pathologic condition.[14,15]

RISK FACTORS

Multiple risk factors for urinary incontinence have been identified. For women, high parity, history of vaginal deliveries, and menopause are risk factors for the development of urinary incontinence.[16–18] Similarly, men who have undergone prostate surgery may be higher risk for incontinence. In both cases, damage to neural control of the bladder or pelvic floor muscles or direct mechanical trauma to the pelvic floor is thought to underlay the development of urinary incontinence.[19] Obesity and increasing age are risk factors for both genders in the development of urinary incontinence.[16–18] After age 80, both genders are equally affected by urinary incontinence.[20]

DIAGNOSIS

The diagnosis of urinary incontinence can be readily made by a physician simply by asking if the patient is experiencing episodes of unintended loss of urine. Because the condition is often embarrassing for patients, individuals may not report incontinence unless directly asked by a physician. Once a diagnosis of urinary incontinence has been made, however, the physician must perform a more thorough history to accurately assess the underlying cause or type of incontinence.

An appropriate history for a patient with urinary incontinence should include an assessment of reversible causes. The DIAPPERS mnemonic created by Resnick provides an easy way to remember the common reversible causes of incontinence, which include:

- D: Delirium
- I: Infection

- A: Atrophic vaginitis
- P: Pharmaceuticals, such as alpha-adrenergic antagonists, ACE inhibitors, calcium channel blockers, diuretics, COX 2 selective NSAIDS, opioids, skeletal muscle relaxants, antidepressants, antipsychotics, alcohol, antihistamines, anticholinergics, and thiazolidinediones.[21,22]
- P: Psychological disorders, such as depression
- E: Excessive urine output secondary to overconsumption of fluids, medications, or chronic conditions, such as diabetes
- R: Reduced mobility
- S: Stool impaction[23]

Once reversible causes have been excluded, the physician must determine the type of urinary incontinence that the patient is experiencing. Eliciting typical symptoms and triggers can help to categorize the type of incontinence. Standardized questionnaires may simplify the process of determining type of incontinence. The 3 Incontinence Questions, for example, has been shown to have a sensitivity of 0.86 for stress incontinence and 0.75 for detecting urge incontinence in middle-aged and older women.[24]

A physician should also consider how other medical and surgical history may contribute to incontinence episodes. For instance, a patient with stress incontinence and chronic cough secondary to chronic obstructive pulmonary disease (COPD) may benefit most from treating the COPD to decrease coughing-triggered incontinence.

In addition to a thorough history, a physical examination focused on anatomic abnormalities and evidence of contributing causes may be helpful in determining the type of incontinence the patient is experiencing.[21,25] The physical examination should include a prostate or gynecologic examination to help rule out contributing causes.[26] If a diagnosis of stress incontinence is suspected, the physician should perform the cough stress test to confirm the diagnosis.[14,27,28] While in the dorsal lithotomy position with a full bladder, a patient is asked to relax his or her pelvic muscles and cough once during the cough stress test. If no leakage occurs, the test should be repeated with the patient in a standing position. A positive test, defined as leaking within 5 to 15 seconds after coughing, confirms the diagnosis of stress incontinence.[22,29,30]

Laboratory studies are not routinely indicated unless the history or physical examination suggests a specific cause, such as polyuria secondary to diabetes. Nonetheless, many physicians find it helpful to obtain a urinalysis and a serum creatinine test to rule out urinary retention, infection, and other reversible causes.[21]

Requesting patient-completed voiding diaries may help a physician to determine patterns or triggers associated with a particular type of incontinence. For example, patients with urge incontinence frequently report awakening 2 or more times per night to void, whereas those with stress incontinence rarely report nighttime symptoms.[31,32] A voiding diary should include a record of all incontinent episodes as well as all continent voiding episodes over a period of time. Three days of record should be sufficient to aid with diagnosis and treatment plans.[33–35]

Although imaging need not be ordered for every patient, if a physician suspects a patient has overflow incontinence, a postvoid residual may be helpful in confirming the diagnosis.[36] A postvoid residual volume may be calculated after the patient has emptied his or her bladder using either ultrasound or intermittent bladder catheterization to quantify the amount of urine remaining in the bladder.[27] A postvoid residual volume of greater than 200 mL is diagnostic of overflow incontinence, whereas a residual volume of less than 50 mL rules out overflow incontinence as a contributor to a patient's symptoms.[21]

TREATMENT

Treatment of urinary incontinence may include lifestyle modifications, medication, or surgical intervention. Treatment recommendations vary by type of urinary incontinence, yet treatment of all types focuses primarily on improved quality of life for the patient rather than disease-oriented outcomes. Thus, treatment modalities should be chosen based on patient preference.[2,21] For all patients with urinary incontinence, psychological intervention should be considered because it may help to improve coping skills and overall quality of life.[37]

Urge Incontinence

Patients with urge incontinence often cite urinary frequency, urgency, and nocturia as the most bothersome symptoms experienced.[20] Depending on the most concerning symptom, patients may use behavioral modifications, medications, devices, or surgery to help alleviate concerns.[38]

Behavioral or lifestyle modifications have been shown to improve urinary incontinence. Initial interventions should include modification of fluid intake and avoidance of bladder irritants, such as caffeine, alcohol, and artificial sweeteners.[39] Encouraging timed voiding every 1 to 2 hours can also greatly improve urge incontinence symptoms.[39] In addition, bladder retraining and pelvic floor muscle strengthening exercises have been shown to be beneficial for patients.[40] When performed properly, pelvic floor muscle exercises have been shown to be more effective than medications for reducing urge incontinence episodes.[41]

Pelvic floor muscle strengthening relies on the repetitive and selective contraction of specific muscles to improve strength, endurance, and muscle coordination, allowing the patient to improve voiding control and delay voiding to allow sufficient time to toilet.[42] Patients may seek out specialized physical therapists to aid in teaching effective muscle strengthening regimens. Furthermore, biofeedback and electrical or magnetic stimulation may also be added to training to allow for optimal improvement in muscle control.[42,43] Some studies have even shown benefit in referring at-risk patients for pelvic floor muscle training in the immediate and late postpartum period to prevent future incontinence.[44]

Although medication alone rarely eradicates urge incontinence episodes, pharmacologic treatment can be an important component in a comprehensive plan to improve incontinence.[20,45] Anticholinergic medications are the preferred first-line pharmaceutical agents for urge incontinence because they reduce detrusor overactivity by antagonizing the M2 and M3 muscarinic receptors in the bladder.[46] Common anticholinergic medications are listed in **Table 1**. Anticholinergic medications should be used by patients for 4 to 8 weeks to accurately ascertain the benefit of the therapy.[38] Unfortunately, side effects, such as tachycardia, palpitations, nausea, constipation, blurry vision, confusion, dry mouth, and urinary retention, are common. Physicians should recommend long-acting anticholinergic medications, such as fesoterodine, oxybutynin, tolterodine, trospium, darifenacin, and solifenacin, to help limit side effects.[38] Patients with narrow angle glaucoma and gastrointestinal obstruction should not use anticholinergic medications.[46] Furthermore, although 60% to 70% of patients in nursing homes have urinary incontinence, anticholinergic medications should be used with caution in this population because of worsening confusion and interaction between anticholinergic medications and cholinesterase inhibitors commonly used to treat dementia.[46]

Beta-adrenergic agonist medication, such as mirabegron, that acts on the beta-3 adrenergic receptors of the detrusor muscle to promote relaxation, is also an option

Table 1
Anticholinergic treatment of urge incontinence

Class	Medication	Dose (mg)	Route	Frequency
Nonselective M3	Propantheline (Pro-Banthine)	7.5–30	Oral	3–5 times daily
	Tolterodine (Detrol LA)	4	Oral	Daily
	Trospium (Sanctura)	20	Oral	2 times daily
	Solifenacin (VESIcare)	5–10	Oral	Daily
Selective M3	Darifenacin (Enablex)	7.5–15	Oral	Daily
Smooth muscle relaxant	Oxybutynin (Ditropan)	2.5–5	Oral	1–3 times daily
	Oxybutynin extended release (Ditropan XL)	5–30	Oral	Daily
	Oxybutynin transdermal (Oxytrol)	4.9	Transdermal	Twice per week
	Hyoscyamine (Levsin)	0.125–0.375	Oral	2–4 times daily

for pharmacologic treatment.[47] When using mirabegron, patients can expect to have 1 to 2 less incontinence episodes per day.[48] Commonly reported side effects with use of mirabegron include nausea, diarrhea, dizziness, headache, and increased blood pressure.[47]

When behavioral and oral pharmacologic interventions have proven ineffective, more invasive treatment modalities may be recommended for urge incontinence. For example, injection of onabotulinumtoxinA into the detrusor muscle may decrease incontinence and improve quality of life, as reported by patients on standardized questionnaires, for 3 to 6 months.[49] Similarly, posterior tibial nerve stimulators may be placed during an in-office procedure and can reduce incontinence in up to 75% of patients who have failed behavioral modification treatment.[38,50] Also, surgery to implant sacral, paraurethral, or pudendal nerve stimulators may also have a role in treatment of refractory urge incontinence.[51]

Stress Incontinence

Whereas urge incontinence results from an overactivity of the detrusor muscle, stress incontinence is the result of a weakening of the urinary sphincter, allowing leakage of urine that is exacerbated by increased intra-abdominal pressure. Lifestyle interventions have been shown to be effective for treatment of both types of incontinence. Weight loss and increased physical activity have been shown to decrease frequency of incontinence symptoms.[39,52] Pilates, yoga, Tai chi, and core training may be particularly helpful for incontinence symptoms.[53] Complementary therapies, such as acupuncture, hypnotherapy, and reflexology, have also been shown to have some benefit.[54–56] Patients should also be educated on managing fluid intake and coordinating intake with toileting schedule to facilitate fewer incontinence episodes.[39] Elimination of contributing factors, such as treatment of constipation and chronic cough, can also help to decrease stress incontinence episodes.[39] Although the mechanism is not well understood, smoking cessation is effective for improving incontinence of both the stress and the urge type.[39]

Although lifestyle changes should be recommended for both urge and stress incontinence patients, no medications are approved for the treatment of stress incontinence. Alpha-adrenergic agonists, such as pseudoephedrine, may have some benefit, although significant adverse effects limit practical usefulness.[57] However, some patients may benefit from taking an alpha-adrenergic agonist twice daily or 1 hour before exercise.[57] Similarly, Cymbalta has been shown to have some benefit in reducing stress incontinence episodes, but adverse effects also limit its off-label use in practice for only stress incontinence as an indication.[58]

Although few pharmacologic options exist for stress incontinence, mechanical devices may prove quite effective for patients as part of a treatment regimen. Intraurethral plugs and extraurethral seals may be fitted that can prevent leakage, whereas pessaries may be used to support the bladder neck and thereby stop stress incontinence events.[59] Pessaries have been shown to be low risk, low cost, and rapidly effective and to have minimal contraindications for patients.[38]

Surgical intervention is often viewed as a last resort in treatment of urinary incontinence because of potential complications of an invasive procedure. However, for stress incontinence, surgery may prove to be quite beneficial and may be a first-line treatment. Ultimately, 30% of women with stress incontinence will choose to undergo surgery.[60] Surgery can be expected to improve incontinence symptoms for many women with improvement rates as high as 90% noted in some studies with complication rates of less than 5%.[2]

Interestingly, stress incontinence treatments have not often been compared in head-to-head effectiveness trials, so physicians should use clinical judgment and patient preference to help guide recommendations for treatment modality to individual patients.[38]

Mixed Incontinence

Mixed incontinence should be treated with strategies for stress and urge incontinence using patient-reported predominant symptoms as a guide for which treatment to use first. Of note, patients with mixed incontinence who undergo surgical treatment of stress incontinence often experience improvement in urge symptoms as well.

Overflow Incontinence

Overflow incontinence occurs when the bladder is unable to empty effectively resulting in overfilling of the bladder with subsequent spillover incontinence. Treatments therefore focus on targeting the underlying pathologic condition contributing to bladder ineffectiveness to facilitate bladder emptying. If medications are causing bladder ineffectiveness, such as occurs with anticholinergic therapies, then those medications should be tapered or discontinued.[38] If neurologic disease has resulted in impaired detrusor innervation, then intermittent or indwelling catheter placement will be the most effective treatment strategy.[38]

Functional Incontinence

Functional incontinence results not from pathologic condition within the genitourinary system, but rather from an ailment that results in cognitive or motor difficulty that leads to the inability for the patient to reach the toilet in a timely appropriate manner. Treatment focuses on assisting with toileting to ensure that the bladder is emptied regularly.[38]

Referral

Physicians in primary care should consider referral of patients to a urologist or urogynecologist when incontinence symptoms are associated with recurrent symptomatic urinary tract infections, new-onset neurologic symptoms, marked prostate enlargement, or pelvic organ prolapse past the introitus. Significant pelvic pain, persistent hematuria, persistent proteinuria, previous pelvic radiation, a postvoid residual greater than 200 mL, or uncertain diagnosis should also prompt referral.[30,61]

REFERENCES

1. Fantl AJ. Urinary incontinence in adults: acute and chronic management/urinary incontinence in adults. Guideline panel update. Rockville (MD): U.S. Department of Health and Human Services; 1996. Agency for Health Care Policy and Research; Clinical Practice Guideline Number 2: AHCPR publication no. 96-0682.
2. Lukacz ES, Santiago-Lastra Y, Albo ME, et al. Urinary incontinence in women: a review. JAMA 2017;318(16):1592–604.
3. Melville JL, Fan MY, Rau H, et al. Major depression and urinary incontinence in women: temporal associations in an epidemiologic sample. Am J Obstet Gynecol 2009;201(490):e1–7.
4. Bogner HR, Gallo JJ, Sammel MD, et al. Urinary incontinence and psychological distress in community-dwelling older adults. J Am Geriatr Soc 2002;50(3): 489–95.
5. Hunskaar S, Burgio K, Clark A, et al. Epidemiology of urinary and faecal incontinence and pelvic organ prolapse. In: Abrams P, Cardozo L, Khoury R, et al, editors. Incontinence. 3rd international consultation on incontinence. Plymouth (United Kingdom): Health Publication Ltd; 2005. p. 255–312.
6. Albertson M. Decreasing urinary incontinence in home healthcare. Home Healthc Now 2018;36(4):232–7.
7. Lin KY, Siu KC, Lin KH. Impact of lower urinary tract symptoms on work productivity in female workers: a systematic review and meta-analysis. Neurourol Urodyn 2018;37(8):2323–34.
8. National Institute for Healthcare and Excellence. The management of urinary incontinence in women. NICE clinical guideline 171 2013.
9. Haylen R, de Ridder D, Freeman R, et al. An International Urogynecological Association (IUGA)/International Continence Society (ICS) joint report on the terminology of female pelvic floor dysfunction. Neurourol Urodyn 2010;29(1):4–20.
10. DuBeau CE, Kuchel GA, Johnson T II, et al. Fourth international consultation on incontinence. Incontinence in the frail elderly: report from the 4th international consultation on incontinence. Neurourol Urodyn 2010;29(1):165–78.
11. Milsom I, Altman D, Cartwright R, et al. Epidemiology of urinary incontinence (UI) and other lower urinary tract symptoms (LUTS), pelvic organ prolapse (POP) and anal incontinence (AI). Incontinence. ICUD-EAU, 2013.
12. Ouslander JG. Management of overactive bladder. N Engl J Med 2004;350(8): 786–99.
13. Schimpf MO, Patel M, O'Sullivan DM, et al. Difference in quality of life in women with urge urinary incontinence compared to women with stress urinary incontinence. Int Urogynecol J Pelvic Floor Dysfunct 2009;20(7):781–6.
14. Holroyd-Leduc JM, Tannenbaum C, Thorpe KE, et al. What type of urinary incontinence does this woman have? JAMA 2008;299(12):1446–56.
15. Yap P, Tan D. Urinary incontinence in dementia - a practical approach. Aust Fam Physician 2006;35(4):237–41.
16. MacArthur C, Lewis M, Bick D. Stress incontinence after childbirth. Br J Midwifery 1993;1(5):207–15.
17. Wilson PD, Herbison RM, Herbison GP. Obstetric practice and the prevalence of urinary incontinence three months after delivery. Br J Obstet Gynaecol 1996; 103(2):154–61.
18. Thom DH, van den Eeden SK, Brown JS. Evaluation of parturition and other reproductive variables as risk factors for urinary incontinence in later life. Obstet Gynecol 1997;90(6):983–9.

19. Glazener CMA, Cooper K. Anterior vaginal repair for urinary incontinence in women. Cochrane Database Syst Rev 2001;(1):CD001755.
20. Gibbs CF, Johnson TM II, Ouslander JG. Office management of geriatric urinary incontinence. Am J Med 2007;120(3):211–20.
21. Weiss BD. Diagnostic evaluation of urinary incontinence in geriatric patients. Am Fam Physician 1998;57(11):2675–84.
22. Imam KA. The role of the primary care physician in the management of bladder dysfunction. Rev Urol 2004;6(suppl 1):S38–44.
23. Resnick NM, Yalla SV. Management of urinary incontinence in the elderly. N Engl J Med 1985;313(13):800–5.
24. Brown JS, Bradley CS, Subak LL, et al, Diagnostic Aspects of Incontinence Study (DAISy) Research Group. The sensitivity and specificity of a simple test to distinguish between urge and stress urinary incontinence. Ann Intern Med 2006; 144(10):715–23.
25. Frank C, Szlanta A. Office management of urinary incontinence among older patients. Can Fam Physician 2010;56(11):1115–20.
26. Chapple CR, Manassero F. Urinary incontinence in adults. Surgery 2005;23(3): 101–7.
27. Culligan PJ, Heit M. Urinary incontinence in women: evaluation and management. Am Fam Physician 2000;62(11):2433–44, 2447, 2452.
28. Videla FL, Wall LL. Stress incontinence diagnosed without multichannel urodynamic studies. Obstet Gynecol 1998;91(6):965–8.
29. Ghoniem G, Stanford E, Kenton K, et al. Evaluation and outcome measures in the treatment of female urinary stress incontinence: International Urogynecological Association (IUGA) guidelines for research and clinical practice. Int Urogynecol J Pelvic Floor Dysfunct 2008;19(1):5–33.
30. Weidner AC, Myers ER, Visco AG, et al. Which women with stress incontinence require urodynamic evaluation? Am J Obstet Gynecol 2001;184(2):20–7.
31. Moore KN, Saltmarche B, Query A. Urinary incontinence. Non-surgical management by family physicians. Can Fam Physician 2003;49:602–10.
32. Wyman JF, Choi SC, Harkins SW, et al. The urinary diary in evaluation of incontinent women: a test-retest analysis. Obstet Gynecol 1988;71(6 pt 1):812–7.
33. Homma Y, Ando T, Yoshida M, et al. Voiding and incontinence frequencies: variability of diary data and required diary length. Neurourol Urodyn 2002;21(3): 204–9.
34. Nygaard I, Holcomb R. Reproducibility of the seven-day voiding diary in women with stress urinary incontinence. Int Urogynecol J Pelvic Floor Dysfunct 2000; 11(1):15–7.
35. Yap TL, Cromwell DC, Emberton M. A systematic review of the reliability of frequency-volume charts in urological research and its implications for the optimum chart duration. BJU Int 2007;99(1):9–16.
36. Dowling-Castronovo A, Specht JK. How to try this: assessment of transient urinary incontinence in older adults. Am J Nurs 2009;109(2):62–71.
37. Shinohara K, Honyashiki M, Imai H, et al. Behavioural therapies versus other psychological therapies for depression. Cochrane Database Syst Rev 2013;(10):CD008696.
38. Hersh L, Salzman B. Clinical management of urinary incontinence in women. Am Fam Physician 2013;87(9):634–40.
39. Imamura M, Williams K, Wells M, et al. Lifestyle interventions for the treatment of urinary incontinence in adults. Cochrane Database Syst Rev 2015;(12):CD003505.

40. Khan IJ, Tariq SH. Urinary incontinence: behavioral modification therapy in older adult. Clin Geriatr Med 2004;20(3):499–509.
41. Burgio KL, Locher JL, Goode PS, et al. Behavioral vs drug treatment for urge urinary incontinence in older women: a randomized controlled trial. JAMA 1998; 280(23):1995–2000.
42. Dumoulin C, Hay-Smith EJC, Mac Habée-Séguin G. Pelvic floor muscle training versus no treatment, or inactive control treatments, for urinary incontinence in women. Cochrane Database Syst Rev 2014;(5):CD005654.
43. McClurg D, Pollock A, Campbell P, et al. Conservative interventions for urinary incontinence in women: an overview of Cochrane systematic reviews. Cochrane Database Syst Rev 2016;(9):CD012337.
44. Saboia DM, Bezerra KC, Vasconcelos Neto JA, et al. The effectiveness of postpartum interventions to prevent urinary incontinence: a systematic review. Rev Bras Enferm 2018;71(suppl 3):1460–8.
45. Norton P, Brubaker L. Urinary incontinence in women. Lancet 2006;367(9504): 57–67.
46. DeMaagd G. Urinary incontinence: treatment update with a focus on pharmacological management. US Pharm 2007;32(6):34–44.
47. Mirabegron (Myrbetriq) for overactive bladder. Med Lett Drugs Ther 2013; 55(1409):13–5.
48. Sacco E, Bientinesi R. Mirabegron: a review of recent data and its prospects in the management of overactive bladder. Ther Adv Urol 2012;4(6):315–24.
49. Duthie JB, Vincent M, Herbison GP, et al. Botulinum toxin injections for adults with overactive bladder syndrome. Cochrane Database Syst Rev 2011;(12):CD005493.
50. Peters KM, Macdiarmid SA, Wooldridge LS, et al. Randomized trial of percutaneous tibial nerve stimulation versus extended-release tolterodine: results from the overactive bladder innovative therapy trial. J Urol 2009;182(3):1055–61.
51. Bosch JL. Electrical neuromodulatory therapy in female voiding dysfunction. BJU Int 2006;98(suppl 1):43–8.
52. Wing RR, West DS, Grady D, et al, Program to Reduce Incontinence by Diet and Exercise Group. Effect of weight loss on urinary incontinence in overweight and obese women: results at 12 and 18 months. J Urol 2010;184(3):1005–10.
53. Bø K, Herbert R. There is not yet strong evidence that exercise regimens other than pelvic floor muscle training can reduce stress urinary incontinence in women: a systematic review. J Physiother 2013;59(3):159–68.
54. Wang Y, Zhishun L, Peng W, et al. Acupuncture for stress urinary incontinence in adults. Cochrane Database Syst Rev 2013;(7):CD009408.
55. Komesu YM, Sapien RE, Rogers RG, et al. Hypnotherapy for treatment of overactive bladder: a randomized controlled trial pilot study. Female Pelvic Med Reconstr Surg 2011;17(6):308–13.
56. Yau K, Mak HL, Cheon WC, et al. Effects of foot reflexology on patients with symptomatic idiopathic detrusor overactivity. Int Urogynecol J Pelvic Floor Dysfunct 2006;18(6):653–8.
57. Alhasso A, Glazener CM, Pickard R, et al. Adrenergic drugs for urinary incontinence in adults. Cochrane Database Syst Rev 2005;(3):CD001842.
58. Mariappan P, Ballantyne Z, N'Dow JM, et al. Serotonin and nor-adrenaline reuptake inhibitors (SNRI) for stress urinary incontinence in adults. Cochrane Database Syst Rev 2005;(3):CD004742.
59. Lipp A, Shaw C, Glavind K. Mechanical devices for urinary incontinence in women. Cochrane Database Syst Rev 2014;(12):CD001756.

60. Dmochowski RR, Blaivas JM, Gormley EA, et al. Female stress urinary incontinence update panel of the American Urological Association Education and Research, Inc. Update of AUA guideline on the surgical management of female stress urinary incontinence. J Urol 2010;183(5):1906–14.
61. Cefalu CA. Urinary incontinence. In: Ham RJ, editor. Primary care geriatrics: a case-based approach. 5th edition. Philadelphia: Mosby Elsevier; 2007. p. 306–23.

Nocturnal Enuresis

Robin A. Walker, MD[a,b,*]

KEYWORDS

• Primary care • Urology • Enuresis • Treatment

KEY POINTS

- Enuresis is a common complaint that presents in the primary care setting.
- It is important to rule out secondary causes of enuresis; however, most cases are considered primary.
- Most children that experience enuresis will not have symptoms that progress past adolescence.
- Medications can help to control symptoms while the child is in the process of developing out of primary enuresis.

DEFINITION, EPIDEMIOLOGY, AND CLASSIFICATION

Enuresis is defined as inappropriate, nonvoluntary discharge of urine past the age of usual control, which is considered to be a developmental age of 5 to 7 years.[1,2] Although studies vary, it is estimated that around 25% of 5-year-old children have episodes of nocturnal enuresis. That rate decreases to less than 10% by the age of 7 owing to a spontaneous annual cure rate of around 15%. Of all children who do experience nocturnal enuresis, only roughly 2% will carry symptoms over into adulthood. The male:female ratio is approximately 3:1. In all, 5 to 7 million children in the United States experience nocturnal enuresis.[3–6]

Enuresis can be characterized in 2 predominant ways in an effort to better understand its causes and how to best treat each patient. These differentiations are primary versus secondary, and monosymptomatic versus polysymptomatic. Primary nocturnal enuresis occurs when the child has never had a period of nighttime dryness that lasts longer than 6 months and this classification accounts for roughly 80% of cases. Secondary nocturnal enuresis occurs when nonvoluntary discharge of urine returns after at least a 6-month period of nighttime dryness, and these cases account for the remaining 20%.[7] When a patient has monosymptomatic enuresis, the only

Disclosure Statement: The author has nothing to disclose.
[a] Department of Family and Community Medicine, University of Kansas School of Medicine–Wichita, 1010 North Kansas, Wichita, KS 67214, USA; [b] Wesley Family Medicine Residency Program, Wichita, KS 67214, USA
* Northwest Family Physicians, 3730 North Ridge Road Suite 100, Wichita, KS 67205.
E-mail address: robin.walker@wesleymc.com

Prim Care Clin Office Pract 46 (2019) 243–248
https://doi.org/10.1016/j.pop.2019.02.005
0095-4543/19/

symptom present is involuntary loss of urine. Polysymptomatic enuresis, however, indicates that the patient has at least 1 additional lower urinary tract symptom such as urgency, frequency, dysuria, or dribbling.[2]

ETIOLOGY AND PATHOPHYSIOLOGY

Primary nocturnal enuresis is caused by a failure to arouse from sleep despite receiving stimuli combined with either excessive urine production, a small capacity of the bladder, or detrusor overactivity.[8] There is a genetic predisposition to primary nocturnal enuresis, with research pointing toward potential loci on chromosomes 12, 13, and 21 as genetic sources. If 1 parent suffered from enuresis as a child, then their offspring have a 44% chance of experiencing enuresis. That number increases to 77% when both parents experienced enuresis. When neither parent was affected, the incidence is 15%.[9–11]

Secondary nocturnal enuresis is caused by either the new onset of a medical condition, such as urinary infection, obstructive sleep apnea, diabetes insipidus, diabetes mellitus, hypothyroidism, and renal disease, or by a new psychological stress. Examples of causes of secondary enuresis are listed in **Table 1** along with associated symptoms they may present with.[12–14]

INITIAL EVALUATION

Elements of the History and Physical

A detailed history and physical examination should be performed with the goal of identifying any signs or symptoms of an underlying organic medical condition. This information is especially important when evaluating for secondary enuresis. Clues can be obtained by paying attention to the onset and frequency, any associated lower urinary tract symptoms, volume of first morning void, soundness of sleep, and by obtaining a detailed family history of nocturnal enuresis. Asking about any potential sources of psychological stress is especially important when evaluating a patient for secondary nocturnal enuresis.

The physical examination of patients with monosymptomatic nocturnal enuresis is usually normal. The physical examination may show evidence of other underlying medical conditions for patients with polysymptomatic or secondary enuresis. Pay

Table 1
Secondary enuresis

Secondary Cause of Enuresis	Associated Symptoms/Clinical Features	Daytime Symptoms
Constipation	Encopresis, hard stools, overflow incontinence	Yes
Urinary tract infection	Urinary frequency, fever, urgency	Yes
Urinary tract dysfunction/malformation	Frequent urinary tract infections	Yes
Overactive bladder	Frequency, urgency, dribbling, incomplete emptying of bladder	Yes
Neurogenic bladder	Incomplete emptying of bladder, difficulty starting stream	Yes
Diabetes mellitus	Polyuria, polydipsia	Yes
Obstructive sleep apnea	Daytime somnolence, snoring	No

attention to the growth chart, presence of elevated blood pressure, tonsillar hypertrophy, abnormal abdominal examination, or abnormality of the lumbar spine.

Laboratory and Imaging Studies

Outside of a simple urinalysis, obtaining routine laboratory or imaging studies is of low yield. Allow the components of the history and physical examination as well as the results of the urinalysis to guide decision making with regard to obtaining additional studies. These additional tests may include an assessment of renal function, polysomnography, evaluation of the anatomy of the lower urinary tract system, and postvoid residual.[13,14]

TREATMENT APPROACH

We focus on the treatment of monosymptomatic primary enuresis, because the treatment of secondary and polysymptomatic enuresis entails addressing the underlying medical condition or psychological stress that is the cause of the patient's symptomology.

The treatment plan for each child should have a foundation of compassion and support from the parents or guardians as well as the physician. Behavioral intervention is most effective in a motivated and cooperative child and, as such, should generally be used in children of a developmental age of 6 and older. If the child is not distressed by the incidents of enuresis, then intervention may need to be delayed until they are internally motivated to participate in treatment.[13,15]

Parents should understand that enuresis is a nonvolitional problem and should be reassured that nearly all cases resolve with time. The discussion with parents should also help to define the goals of treatment. These goals can range from short-term dryness for an event (sleeping away from home at camp or a relative or friend's home), decreased impact of enuresis on the child and family, a decrease in the number of wet nights, or prevention of recurrence once dryness has occurred.[13,16,17]

Behavioral Interventions

It is essential to avoid words or actions that instill shame, guilt, or blame. Enuresis occurs outside of the child's control; therefore, punishing the child when events occur is counterproductive and parents should be prepared with a plan for how they will address wet events without emotion when they do occur.[18] Involving a child in the clean-up can be appropriate; however, this should be done with an attitude of sharing in the responsibility and not as a punishment.

Simple behavioral strategies include encouraging the child to empty his or her bladder frequently during the day and before bedtime, limiting fluid intake in the evening, and avoiding caffeinated beverages. Additionally, setting an alarm to awake the child to urinate during the night is an appropriate strategy. Reward systems can help to reinforce positive behavior; however, rewards should be based on the actions that the child can control and not on those that are out of their control. Keeping a calendar of wet and dry nights can help to track the success of interventions, but again caution should be used when considering using the calendar as a basis for rewards.[2,17]

Bed Alarm Therapy

Enuretic alarms are considered a first-line treatment for monosymptomatic nocturnal enuresis, especially when associated with small bladder size or nocturnal detrusor overactivity.[2,19] They have been shown to be as effective as desmopressin with a low relapse rate.[19] When the sensor in the nightclothes or bedding gets wet, the alarm is activated, which startles the child, improving arousal from sleep. After awakening, the child should be encouraged to finish voiding in the toilet. Afterward, the child returns to the room, participates in the change of the bedding and underwear, and resets the alarm after cleaning the sensor or replacing it if it is disposable. Initially, the parent may need to help awaken the child when the alarm sounds. Alarms should be continued until there is a period of 14 consecutive dry nights. This response can take anywhere from 5 to 24 weeks, with most children responding between 12 and 16 weeks.[20]

Pharmacotherapy

Desmopressin is taken in the early evening to decrease urine production and is considered a first-line treatment for children who do not respond to behavioral interventions alone or for those who need an immediate response (ie, sleeping away from home).[2] Desmopressin works by inducing a profound antidiuretic effect without causing any pressor activity. The medication increases the reabsorption of fluid from the renal tubules, thereby decreasing urine production. Eighty percent of patients have a good response rate; however, there is a high incidence of recurrence, with cessation with some studies showing that this rate approaches 65%.[21] It is reasonable to try tapering the dose every 3 months, and studies show that a gradual decrease of the dose can greatly reduce the relapse rate.[22]

Oxybutynin, an anticholinergic and antispasmodic agent that decreases detrusor muscle contractions, is not typically effective as monotherapy in patients with monosymptomatic nocturnal enuresis. It can, however, be added to desmopressin in children who experience daytime incontinence owing to urgency as well as in patients who do not respond to desmopressin alone.[23,24]

The tricyclic medication imipramine is approved by the US Food and Drug Administration for the treatment of nocturnal enuresis. It works by decreasing REM time, stimulating antidiuretic hormone secretion, and relaxing detrusor muscle. It does have significant side effects (anxiety, dizziness, drowsiness, lethargy, dry mouth, anorexia, vomiting) and serious adverse effects (hepatotoxicity and cardiotoxicity). Imipramine should be used in patients who have failed to respond to other therapies.[2,23,25] On average, it reduces wet nights by 1 event per week and was similarly affective as desmopressin. Upon discontinuation, the relapse rate for patients treated with imipramine alone has been observed to be as high as 96%.[23]

Alternative therapies such as acupuncture, hypnosis, psychotherapy, herbal remedies, and chiropractic manipulation have shown modest benefit in small studies and are not considered routine interventions.[26]

Failure of a child to respond to adequate therapy, defined by a decrease of 50% in the frequency of wet events, should raise suspicions for potential secondary causes. Additional laboratory and imaging studies may be warranted and should be considered. Referral to a provider who specializes in bedwetting should be considered in refractory cases as well.

SUMMARY

Nocturnal enuresis is a common problem that children may present with in a primary care setting. It is important to take a detailed history to rule out potential secondary causes; however, most cases are primary in nature. It is essential to demystify the problem and reassure parents by educating them that the episodes are nonvolitional and the vast majority of children grow out of the problem over time. Behavioral interventions are considered first line and are most successful when the child is invested in succeeding with nighttime dryness. Interventions should be initiated with specific goals in mind. Enuresis alarms are effective and should be considered a first-line intervention for most children. Medications, especially desmopressin, are effective and should be used in conjunction with behavioral interventions.

REFERENCES

1. American Psychiatric Association. Diagnostic and statistical manual of mental disorders, 5th ed., (DSM-5). Washington, DC: American Psychiatric Publishing; 2013.
2. Neveus T, von Gontard A, Hoebeke P, et al. The standardization of terminology of lower urinary tract function in children and adolescents: report from the Standardisation Committee of the International Children's Continence Society. J Urol 2006; 176(1):314–24.
3. Fergusson DM, Horwood LJ, Shannon FT. Factors related to the age of attainment of bladder control: an 8 year longitudinal study. Pediatrics 1986;78(5):884–90.
4. Byrd RS, Weitzman M, Lanphear NE, et al. Bed-Wetting in US children: epidemiology and related behavior problems. Pediatrics 1996;90(3 pt 1):414–9.
5. Butler RJ, Heron J. The prevalence of infrequent bedwetting and nocturnal enuresis in childhood. A large British cohort. Scand J Urol Nephrol 2008;43(3): 257–64.
6. Forsythe WI, Redmond A. Enuresis and spontaneous cure rate. Study of 1129 enuretics. Arch Dis Child 1974;49(4):259.
7. Von Gontard A, Mauer-Muckle K, Plück J, et al. Clinical behavioral problems in day- and night-wetting children. Pediatr Nephrol 1999;13(8):662.
8. Norgaard JP, Djurhuss JC. The pathophysiology of enuresis in children and young adults. Clin Pediatr (Phila) 1993;(Spec No):5–9.
9. Bakwin H. Enuresis in twins. Am J Dis Child 1971;121(3):222.
10. Eiberg H, Berendt I, Mohr J. Assignment of dominant inherited nocturnal enuresis (ENUR1) to chromosome 13q. Nat Genet 1995;10(3):354.
11. Loeys B, Hoebeke P, Raes A, et al. Does monosymptomatic enuresis exist? A molecular genetic exploration of 32 families with enuresis/incontinence. BJU Int 2002;90(1):76.
12. Vande Walle J, Rittig S, Bauer S, et al, American Academy of Pediatrics, European Society for Paediatric Urology, European Society for Paediatric Nephrology, International Children's Continence Society. Practical consensus guidelines for the management of enuresis. Eur J Pediatr 2012;171:971–83.
13. Neveus T, Eggert P, Evans J, et al. Evaluation of and treatment for monosymptomatic enuresis: a standardization document from the International Children's Incontinence Society. J Urol 2010;183:441.
14. Robson WL, Leung AK. Secondary Nocturnal Enuresis. Clin Pediatr (Phila) 2000; 39:379.
15. Glazener SMA, Evans JHC. Simple behavioural and physical interventions for nocturnal enuresis in children. The Cochrane Library 2008 Issue 2. Ed. Chichester (United Kingdom): John Wiley and Sons, Ltd.
16. Kiddoo D. Nocturnal enuresis. BMJ Clin Evid 2007;2007. p. 0305.
17. Schmitt BD. Nocturnal enuresis. Pediatr Rev 1997;18:183.
18. Van Londen A, van Londen-Berensten MW, van Son MJ, et al. Arousal Training for children suffering from nocturnal enuresis: a 2 ½ year follow up. Behav Res Ther 1993;31:316.

19. Glazener CM, Evans JH, Peto RE. Alarm interventions for nocturnal enuresis in children. Cochrane Database Syst Rev 2005;(2):CD002911.
20. Rushton HG. Nocturnal enuresis: epidemiology, evaluation and currently available treatment options. J Pediatr 1989;114:691.
21. Kwak KW, Lee YS, Park KH, et al. Efficacy of desmopressin and enuresis alarms as first and second line treatment for primary monosymptomatic nocturnal enuresis: prospective randomized crossover study. J Urol 2010;184:2521–6.
22. Chua ME, Silangcruz JM, Chang SJ, et al. Desmopressin withdrawal strategy for pediatric enuresis: a meta-analysis. Pediatrics 2016;138 [pii:e20160495].
23. Lee T, Suh HJ, Lee HJ, et al. Comparison of effects of treatment of primary nocturnal enuresis with oxybutynin plus desmopressin, desmopressin alone or imipramine alone: a randomized control trial. J Urol 2005;174:1084–7.
24. Austin PF, Ferguson G, Yan Y, et al. Combination therapy with desmopressin and an anticholinergic medication for nonresponders to desmopressin for monosymptomatic nocturnal enuresis: a randomized double-blind, placebo-controlled trial. Pediatrics 2008;122:1027.
25. Caldwell PH, Sureshkumar P, Wong WC. Tricyclic and related drugs for nocturnal enuresis in children. Cochrane Database Syst Rev 2016;(1):CD002117.
26. Huang T, Shu X, Huang YS, et al. Complementary and miscellaneous interventions for nocturnal enuresis in children. Cochrane Database Syst Rev 2011;(12):CD005230.

Erectile Dysfunction

Gretchen M. Irwin, MD, MBA

KEYWORDS

• Erectile dysfunction • Phosphodiesterase 5 inhibitor medication • Cardiac disease

KEY POINTS

- Erectile dysfunction is common but undertreated, because of patient reluctance to self-report.
- Patients with cardiac disease, hypertension, hyperlipidemia, and diabetes should be screened for erectile dysfunction.
- Patients with erectile dysfunction may have undiagnosed diabetes or cardiac disease and should be evaluated for these conditions.
- Oral medications can be used safely and easily by many patients for the treatment of erectile dysfunction, although patient education is critical for effective use.

INTRODUCTION

Erectile dysfunction is defined by the Fourth International Consultation on Sexual Medicine as the consistent or recurrent inability to attain and/or maintain penile erection sufficient for sexual satisfaction.[1] Erectile dysfunction is a common condition, affecting up to 30 million men in the United States.[2] Physicians should ask male patients about sexual health to identify men affected by erectile dysfunction, to identify potentially life-threatening underlying conditions associated with erectile dysfunction, and to improve overall quality of life for the patients.

PATHOPHYSIOLOGY AND RISK FACTORS

Erectile function is dependent on a complex interaction of vascular and neural processes. The internal pudendal artery supplies the majority of the blood flow to the penis through the cavernosal branches whereas venous outflow occurs through a network of easily compressible venules. When arousal occurs, parasympathetic activity from the sacral segments of the spinal cord initiates a cascade of events to release nitric oxide and increase intracellular cyclic guanosine monophosphate. Cyclic guanosine monophosphate increases result in vascular smooth muscle relaxation and

Disclosure: The author has nothing to disclose.

Wichita Family Medicine Residency, Department of Family and Community Medicine, Wesley Medical Center, University of Kansas School of Medicine, 1010 North Kansas, Wichita, KS 67214, USA
E-mail address: gdickson@kumc.edu

Prim Care Clin Office Pract 46 (2019) 249–255
https://doi.org/10.1016/j.pop.2019.02.006 **primarycare.theclinics.com**
0095-4543/19/

an increase in blood flow into the corpora cavernosa. This rapid inflow of blood leads to compression of the venule network to decrease venous outflow, thereby raising intracavernosal pressure and resulting in erection. Erectile dysfunction, therefore, can result from any process that impairs either the neural or vascular pathways that contribute to erection.

Because aging is an independent risk factor for the development of erectile dysfunction, many men assume that sexual impairment is an inevitable consequence of growing older.[3–5] Up to one-third of 70 year old men, however, in a recent study reported no erectile difficulty.[6] Thus, a physician should still perform a thorough history and physical examination to rule out other causes before assuming that new-onset erectile dysfunction is solely the result of advancing age.

Risk factors for developing erectile dysfunction include tobacco use, obesity, sedentary lifestyle, and chronic alcohol use.[3–5] Such risk factors are believed to cause hormonal changes that result in low testosterone and impaired endothelial function, which contribute to the development of erectile dysfunction. Both hypothyroidism and hyperthyroidism also may result in significant hormonal derangements that can result in the development of erectile dysfunction.[7]

Patients who have previously been diagnosed with diabetes mellitus, hypertension, dyslipidemia, or depression also have a higher risk of developing erectile dysfunction.[3–5] Of men diagnosed with erectile dysfunction, approximately 40% have hypertension, 42% have hyperlipidemia, and 20% have diabetes.[8–10]

Medication side effects may account for as many as 25% of all cases of erectile dysfunction. In general, antihypertensives, antidepressants, and antipsychotic medications are most likely to cause impaired erectile function, although the exact mechanism is often not well defined. Specific medications that have been associated with erectile dysfunction include α-blockers, benzodiazepines, β-blockers, clonidine, digoxin, histamine H2-receptor blockers, ketoconazole, methyldopa, monoamine oxidase inhibitors, phenobarbital, phenytoin, selective serotonin reuptake inhibitors, spironolactone, thiazide diuretics, and tricyclic antidepressants. Although chronic diseases, such as diabetes mellitus and hypertension, are considered risk factors for developing erectile dysfunction, erectile dysfunction is a key risk factor for development of cardiovascular and metabolic disease.[11,12] Studies suggest that the degree of erectile dysfunction severity a patient experiences may correlate with cardiovascular disease risk, with erectile dysfunction onset preceding a cardiovascular event by up to 5 years.[13–15] Additionally, patients with erectile dysfunction are more likely to also have premature ejaculation, lower urinary tract symptoms associated with benign prostatic hypertrophy, and overactive bladder compared with the general male population.[9]

DIAGNOSIS

A diagnosis of erectile dysfunction can be readily made by a primary care physician. A patient is unlikely to spontaneously self-report erectile dysfunction, however. Rather, a physician should inquire about erectile dysfunction symptoms in at-risk patients.[16]

Once a patient has reported erectile dysfunction symptoms, a physician must take a careful history to determine the extent of symptoms as well as the contribution to symptoms by associated chronic diseases, medication use, or psychosocial issues. Onset of symptoms, severity, degree of impact on daily life, and situational factors that exacerbate symptoms are critical issues to discuss with patients. Many physicians prefer the use of validated questionnaires to help both diagnose and track treatment effectiveness for patients with erectile dysfunction. Examples of validated questionnaires that may be used include the Erection Hardness Score, Sexual Health Inventory for Men, and International Index of Erectile Function.[17,18] Furthermore, a physician should discuss psychosocial issues with patients, such as current relationship dynamics, individual views of sexuality and sexual function, and current life stressors.[19]

In addition to thorough sexual, past medical, past surgical, medication, and psychosocial histories, a diagnosis of erectile dysfunction requires an appropriate physical examination. A physician should assess pulse, blood pressure, and weight given the association of erectile dysfunction with obesity and hypertension. Patients also should be assessed for signs consistent with testosterone deficiency because low testosterone can contribute to erectile dysfunction and may alter treatment recommendations. Several studies have shown a link between erectile dysfunction and osteoporosis.[20,21] In 1 study, men with erectile dysfunction were noted to have a 3-fold increase in incidence of osteoporosis compared with men without erectile dysfunction, independent of other risk factors, such as diabetes or hypertension.[21] It is believed that low androgens, high inflammation causing endothelial dysfunction, and/or reduced nitric oxide activity may play a role in increased bone reabsorption.[21] Physicians counsel patients about the importance of maintaining good bone health.[20] Laboratory studies are not required to diagnose erectile dysfunction, but, given the association with chronic disease, men with newly diagnosed erectile dysfunction should have a hemoglobin A_{1c} and lipid panel evaluated. Young men who develop erectile dysfunction should be screened for coronary vascular disease because these men may have up to a 50% increase in risk of future cardiac events.[22] A morning testosterone should be obtained, because a result less than 300 mg/dL in the setting of testosterone deficiency symptoms warrants treatment of low testosterone as well as erectile dysfunction. Treating both conditions may have an additive benefit for patients. Emerging evidence suggests that mean platelet volume and platelet distribution width may be elevated in men with diabetes at risk of erectile dysfunction, although routine ordering of platelet studies currently is not recommended.[23]

TREATMENT

Multiple treatment modalities exist for erectile dysfunction. Although patients often start with oral medication therapy, other options, such as a surgically implanted penile prosthesis or intraurethral and intracavernosal therapies, should be discussed with patients at the outset. Patient preferences after a discussion of risks and benefits should guide treatment. Ultimately, the goal of treatment should be to improve patient quality of life by restoring sexual function when possible and improving overall health by mitigating risk factors for cardiac and metabolic disease.

Lifestyle changes should be recommended to all patients. Improved diet to facilitate lower blood pressure and weight loss, increased physical activity, and elimination of tobacco use can improve effectiveness of treatment while decreasing risk of concomitant chronic disease. Treatment of chronic diseases, such as diabetes, hypertension, hyperlipidemia, hypothyroidism, depression, and low testosterone, can improve erectile dysfunction symptoms as well as improve effectiveness of oral medication treatment of erectile dysfunction.[7] Improved blood pressure control has been demonstrated to improve erectile dysfunction symptoms as well as decrease men's risk of acquiring erectile dysfunction.[24] The impact of treatment of metabolic disease should not be underestimated because treatment with 40 mg of simvastatin for 6 months significantly improved sexual health related quality of life for men over age 40 years with untreated erectile dysfunction.[25]

Many patients elect to treat erectile dysfunction with oral medications. Approved medications include 4 phosphodiesterase type 5 (PDE5) inhibitors, namely sildenafil, tadalafil, vardenafil, and avanafil. Each medication works by inhibiting the PDE5 enzyme action on cyclic guanosine monophosphate. Erection hardness and duration increase with accumulation of cyclic guanosine monophosphate in the penile cavernosa. Men with disrupted penile vasculature will not benefit from PDE5 inhibitor medications.

Medication interactions are an important consideration before prescribing PDE5 inhibitor medications to patients. PDE5 inhibitors have been shown to interact with antidepressant, antifungal, antiretroviral, and antihypertensive medications. Undoubtedly, however, the most significant interaction occurs between PDE5 inhibitors and nitrate medications. Concomitant use can result in severe hypotension for patients. Men on chronic nitrate medications should not use PDE5 inhibitors. Men who use occasional sublingual nitrates for treatment of angina should not use the nitrate medication and a PDE5 inhibitor within 24 hours of each other. Although medication interactions should be considered prior to prescribing PDE5 inhibitor medications, the presence of significant cardiac or renal disease alone should not be considered a contraindication for treatment. Men should be healthy enough to engage in sexual intercourse, although even dialysis patients have been shown appropriate candidates for use of PDE5 inhibitor medication.[26]

When prescribing PDE5 inhibitor medications, physicians should consider the differences in onset of action and efficacy to help determine the best choice for an individual patient. Avanafil has the shortest onset of action at 15 minutes to 30 minutes as well as the smallest window of effectiveness, with time of effectiveness at only 6 hours. Sildenafil and vardenafil have similar onsets of action at 30 minutes to 60 minutes, respectively, and similar lengthg of effectiveness at 12 hours and 10 hours, respectively. Both of these medications can be less effective if taken with a high-fat meal. Tadalafil requires 60 minutes to 120 minutes for onset of action but can have effect for up to 36 hours. Tadalafil can be taken daily or on an as-needed basis, although no efficacy benefit has been shown for 1 dosing strategy over the other. In a meta-analysis of 82 trials, 1 report suggests that sildenafil, 50 mg, is most likely to be effective whereas tadalafil, 10 mg, is most tolerable for patients.[27] Treatment should be optimized for individual patients, with a trial of medications and titration of doses to find the best effect for the least side effects. **Table 1** summarizes available medication options.

To increase the effectiveness of oral medications, physicians should ensure that patients have been educated on proper use, including the timing of medication in relation to planned intercourse and to mealtimes. Studies suggest that, of patients who failed oral medication therapy for erectile dysfunction, more than half were successful when given additional education on how to use the medication.[28,29]

Table 1
Medications for use in erectile dysfunction

	Onset of Action	Effectiveness Time	Dosage
Avanafil	15–30 min	6 h	50 mg, 100 mg, or 200 mg, once daily, as needed
Sildenafil	30–60 min	12 h	20 mg, 25 mg, 50 mg, or 100 mg, once daily, as needed
Tadalafil	60–120 min	36 h	10 mg or 20 mg, once daily, as needed, *OR* 2.5 mg or 5 mg daily
Vardenafil	30–60 min	10 h	10 mg or 20 mg once daily, as needed

If men cannot or choose not to take an oral medication, intraurethral or intracavernosal alprostadil may be an option. Alprostadil can be inserted as a pellet via a delivery catheter in the meatus or may be injected into the corpus cavernosa. Although there may be some initial reluctance to use alprostadil delivery systems, many men who do initiate therapy report high satisfaction with the medication. In 1 study of 596 men, the overall satisfaction rate with alprostadil treatment was 78.3%, with 86% of patients willing to recommend alprostadil therapy to friends.[30]

Nonpharmacologic options for treatment of erectile dysfunction include vacuum devices and penile prosthesis. Vacuum devices and prostheses have been shown effective and result in high patient and partner satisfaction. Men who have undergone prostate surgery for prostate cancer or benign prostatic hypertrophy who experience erectile dysfunction may find vacuum devices particularly effective.[31] Investigational treatments include extracorporeal shock wave therapy, intracavernosal stem cell therapy, and platelet-rich plasma therapy.

Erectile dysfunction can be diagnosed and managed by primary care physicians. Patients should be referred, however, to urology for additional diagnostic and treatment interventions when men are young, have a history of pelvic trauma, have failed prior erectile dysfunction therapies, have lifelong erectile dysfunction, or have concomitant Peyronie disease.[32] Referral to cardiology may be warranted in the setting of strong family history or severe personal history of cardiac disease to evaluate if a patient is healthy enough for intercourse and for medical treatment of erectile dysfunction. Many men have either a psychological component that contributes to erectile dysfunction or experience psychological distress as a result of erectile dysfunction. Accordingly, men should be encouraged to seek psychotherapy in additional to medical therapy because several studies have shown outcomes are better with combined therapy than either modality alone.[32,33]

REFERENCES

1. McCabe MP, Sharlip ID, Atalla E, et al. Definitions of sexual dysfunctions in women and men: a consensus statement from the Fourth International Consultation on Sexual Medicine 2015. J Sex Med 2016;13:135.
2. McKinlay JB. The worldwide prevalence and epidemiology of erectile dysfunction. Int J Impot Res 2000;12(suppl 4):S6.
3. Grover SA, Lowensteyn I, Kaouache M, et al. The prevalence of erectile dysfunction in the primary care setting: importance of risk factors for diabetes and vascular disease. Arch Intern Med 2006;166:213.
4. Sasayma S, Ishii N, Ishikura F, et al. Men's health study: epidemiology of erectile dysfunction and cardiovascular disease. Circ J 2003;67:656.
5. Kloner RA. Erectile dysfunction in the cardiac patient. Curr Urol Rep 2003;4:466.
6. Feldman HA, Goldstein I, Hatzichristou DG, et al. Impotence and its medical and psychosocial correlates: results of the Massachusetts Male Aging Study. J Urol 1994;151:54–61.
7. Gabrielson AT, Sartor RA, Hellstrom WJG. The impact of thyroid disease on sexual dysfunction in men and women. Sex Med Rev 2019;7(1):57–70.
8. Selvin E, Burnett AL, Platz EA. Prevalence and risk factors for erectile dysfunction in the US. Am J Med 2007;120:151.
9. Seftel AD, Sun P, Swindle R. The prevalence of hypertension, hyperlipidemia, diabetes mellitus and depression in men with erectile dysfunction. J Urol 2004;171: 2341.

10. Manolis A, Doumas M. Sexual dysfunction the 'prima ballerina' of hypertension related quality of life complications. J Hypertens 2008;26:2074.
11. Saigal CS, Wessells H, Pace J, et al. Predictors and prevalence of erectile dysfunction in a racially diverse population. Arch Intern Med 2006;166:207.
12. Bacon C, Mittleman M, Kawachi I, et al. A prospective study of risk factors for erectile dysfunction. J Urol 2006;176:217.
13. Montsori P, Ravagnani P, Galli S, et al. The triad of endothelial dysfunction, cardiovascular disease and erectile dysfunction: clinical implications. Eur Urol 2009;8:58.
14. Hodges L, Kirby M, Solanki J, et al. The temporal relationship between erectile dysfunction and cardiovascular disease. Int J Clin Pract 2007;61:2019.
15. Montsori P, Briganti A, Salonia A, et al. Erectile dysfunction prevalence, time of onset and association with risk factors in 300 consecutive patients with acute chest pain and angiographically documented coronary artery disease. Eur Urol 2003;44:360.
16. Marwick C. Survey says patients expect little physician help on sex. JAMA 1999; 281:2173.
17. Mulhall J, Goldstein I, Bushmakin A, et al. Validation of the erection hardness score. J Sex Med 2007;4:1626.
18. Rosen R, Cappelleri JC, Smith M, et al. Development and evaluation of an abridged, 5- item version of the International Index of Erectile Function (IIEF-5) as a diagnostic tool for erectile dysfunction. Int J Impot Res 1999;11:319.
19. Corona G, Petrone L, Mannucci E. Assessment of the relationship factor in male patients consulting for sexual dysfunction: the concept of couple sexual dysfunction. J Androl 2006;27:795.
20. Dursun M, Özbek E, Otunctemur A, et al. Possible association between erectile dysfunction and osteoporosis in men. Prague Med Rep 2015;116(1):24–30.
21. Wu CH, Lu YY, Chai CY, et al. Increased risk of osteoporosis in patients with erectile dysfunction: a nationwide population-based cohort study. Medicine (Baltimore) 2016;95(26):e4024.
22. Inman B, Sauver J, Jacobson D, et al. A population based longitudinal study of erectile dysfunction and future coronary artery disease. Mayo Clin Proc 2009; 84:108.
23. El Taieb MA, Hegazy EM, Maklad SM, et al. Platelet Indices as a marker for early prediction of erectile dysfunction in diabetic patients. Andrologia 2019;51: e13163.
24. Cordero A, Bertomeu-Martínez V, Mazón P, et al. Erectile dysfunction may improve by blood pressure control in patients with high-risk hypertension. Postgrad Med 2010;122(6):51–6.
25. Trivedi D, Wellsted DM, Collard JB, et al. Simvastatin improves the sexual health-related quality of life in men aged 40 years and over with erectile dysfunction: additional data from the erectile dysfunction and statin trial. BMC Urol 2014; 14:24.
26. Lasaponara F, Sedigh O, Pasquale G, et al. Phosphodiesterase type 5 inhibitor treatment for erectile dysfunction in patients with end-stage renal disease receiving dialysis or after renal transplantation. J Sex Med 2013;10(11): 2798–814.
27. Chen L, Staubli SE, Schneider MP, et al. Phosphodiesterase 5 inhibitors for the treatment of erectile dysfunction: a trade-off network meta-analysis. Eur Urol 2015;68(4):674–80.

28. Jiann B, Yu C, Su C, et al. Rechallenge prior sildenafil nonresponders. Int J Impot Res 2004;16:64.
29. Gruenwald I, Shenfeld O, Chen J, et al. Positive effect of counseling and dose adjustment in patients with erectile dysfunction who failed treatment with sildenafil. Eur Urol 2006;50:134.
30. Alexandre B, Lemaire A, Desvaux P, et al. Intracavernous injections of prostaglandin E1 for erectile dysfunction: patient satisfaction and quality of sex life on long-term treatment. J Sex Med 2007;4(2):426–31.
31. Brison D, Seftel A, Sadeghi-Nejad H. The resurgence of the vacuum erection device (VED) for treatment of erectile dysfunction. J Sex Med 2013;10(4):1124–35.
32. Burnett A, Nehra A, Breau R, et al. Erectile dysfunction: AUA guideline. J Urol 2018;200(3):633–41.
33. Wylie K, Jones R, Walters S. The potential benefit of vacuum devices augmenting psychosexual therapy for erectile dysfunction: a randomized controlled trial. J Sex Marital Ther 2003;29:227.

Prostate Cancer Screening

James D. Holt, MD*, Fereshteh Gerayli, MD

KEYWORDS

- Prostate cancer • Prostate cancer screening • PSA • PSA screening
- Prostate cancer treatment • Overdiagnosis

KEY POINTS

- The benefits of prostate-specific antigen (PSA) screening in men aged 55 to 69 at average risk for prostate cancer are small: reduced risk for prostate cancer deaths and metastatic disease, but no decrease in overall mortality.
- To realize the benefits from PSA screening in men at average risk for prostate cancer, PSA thresholds must be low enough that many false positives, many biopsies, and overdiagnosis of indolent cancers will occur.
- The harms of PSA screening for prostate cancer are significant: anxiety, complications from biopsy, and morbidity from overly aggressive treatment.
- There is little evidence evaluating benefits of PSA screening in populations at increased risk for prostate cancer, such as men with a positive family history or African American men.
- Men 70 and older experience less benefit and more harm from PSA screening for prostate cancer. PSA screening is not recommended for them.

INTRODUCTION

Prostate cancer is the most common noncutaneous malignancy and the second most common cause of cancer death in men. Prostate cancer is diagnosed in an estimated 233,000 men in the United States each year and causes 29,480 deaths, primarily in men 65 to 79 years old. The lifetime risk for developing prostate cancer is 15.3% in US men.[1]

EVIDENCE REVIEW

Two large randomized controlled trials have examined the risks and benefits of systematic screening of asymptomatic men for prostate cancer. Both the Prostate, Lung, Colorectal, and Ovarian (PLCO) Screening Trial and the European Randomized Study of Screening for Prostate Cancer (ERSPC) have significant flaws, which make them less useful for formulating strong evidence-based guidelines.[2] Accordingly, despite huge populations studied, less is known about the benefits of prostate cancer screening than would be expected.

Disclosure Statement: The authors have nothing to disclose.
Johnson City Family Medicine Residency Program, East Tennessee State University Quillen College of Medicine, ETSU Family Medicine Associates, 917 West Walnut Street, Johnson City, TN 37604-6527, USA
* Corresponding author.
E-mail address: holtj@etsu.edu

Prim Care Clin Office Pract 46 (2019) 257–263
https://doi.org/10.1016/j.pop.2019.02.007

The American trial, the PLCO, compared systematic prostate-specific antigen (PSA) screening with usual care in 76,683 men. However, usual care often included PSA screening and did include PSA measurement in men with prostate symptoms: 78% of the men in the control group had at least one PSA measurement during the study.[2] The screening interval was yearly, and the cutoff value for a positive test was 4.0 ng/mL. PSA screening showed no benefit, neither in the initial study nor with extended follow-up, in reducing prostate cancer deaths or all-cause mortality, in the PLCO Trial. Metastatic prostate cancer was not tracked.

The ERSPC did show a benefit from PSA screening.[2] Of note, each clinical site participating in the ERSPC set its own cutoff PSA value for biopsy as well as its own screening interval. The clinical site in Goteborg, Sweden demonstrated such a strong benefit from PSA screening that the study would not have been positive without including this site.[3] The Goteborg site tested every 2 years, more frequently than most sites, and had the lowest cutoff value, 2.5 ng/dL, of any ERSPC site. The Goteborg site experienced a 42% relative risk (RR) reduction in prostate cancer mortality after 14 years of follow-up.[2] The absolute risk reduction at the Goteborg site was 0.4% over 14 years, that is, 4 fewer men died of prostate cancer in the intervention group per 1000 men screened, over the course of the study. In comparison, the Netherlands site, which was second only to the Swedish site in demonstrating a benefit to PSA screening, demonstrated a 20% RR reduction in prostate cancer mortality after 12.8 years. Most of the ERSPC clinical sites, including the largest site in Finland, did not show a significant reduction in prostate cancer deaths. The study as a whole, however, did show a significant benefit: a 22% RR reduction in prostate cancer mortality. The absolute risk reduction in prostate cancer deaths was 1.28 fewer prostate cancer deaths per 1000 men screened over 13 years.[2]

The other benefit demonstrated in the ERSPC was a reduction in metastatic prostate cancer. Only the sites in Sweden, the Netherlands, Finland, and Switzerland tracked metastatic prostate cancer. Among the men randomized to PSA screening at those sites, which included Goteborg, Sweden, and the Netherlands, the 2 sites showing the greatest reduction in prostate cancer mortality, the risk of developing metastatic prostate cancer was reduced by 30% in men randomized to screening. The absolute risk reduction was 3.1 fewer metastatic cases per 1000 men.[2]

The Cluster Randomized Trial of PSA Testing for Prostate Cancer (CAP Trial) randomized 415,357 men in the United Kingdom to a single PSA screening or no screening between 2001 and 2009. Only 36% of the men randomized to screening were screened, and the investigators estimated 10% to 15% of the control group had at least one PSA level drawn. Although more cases of prostate cancer were identified, there was no mortality benefit from the screening.[4] The CAP Trial was embedded in the ProtecT Trial, which evaluated the various treatment options for PSA-detected prostate cancer.

The Stockholm Trial also randomized men to a single PSA screen in 1988, but enrolled only 2400 men. No significant difference in prostate cancer mortality nor in overall survival was noted.[3]

The Quebec Study, randomizing 46,486 men in Quebec City to ongoing PSA screening or usual care, suffered major methodological problems. For example, there was no way to determine if adequate randomization or blinding was done, and only 23.6% of the men in the intervention group were screened, versus 7.3% of the control group. No difference in prostate cancer mortality was found, using intention-to-screen analysis.[3]

The Norrkoping Study enrolled 9026 men aged 50 to 69 to an intervention group receiving 2 rectal examinations and 2 PSA levels or a control group of usual care. In the intervention group, each screen was about 3 years apart. Of men in the intervention group, 70% to 78% were screened during the 4 screening periods, but the number of controls who received screening was not tracked. No significant difference in prostate cancer mortality nor in overall survival was noted.[3]

There are several other tests for risk stratification after an abnormal PSA, such as urinary and serum biomarkers, imaging, risk calculators, and genomic testing, to identify men who are likely to have prostate cancer and/or one with aggressive phenotypes. However, availability may be limited based on institutional affiliation.[5] In addition, these techniques require more validation in larger patient cohorts and have not been standardized and integrated into usual clinical practice.

DISCUSSION

Unfortunately, even though prostate cancer screening via PSA testing has been studied with several large, well-funded studies, the evidence does not provide a clear recommendation to screen or not to screen.[2] There certainly are trends, which should direct current guidelines for screening, but researchers still have not produced definitive evidence.

PSA screening leads to overdiagnosis (ie, diagnosis of prostate cancer in men who have indolent cancers, which otherwise would never come to clinical notice) and overtreatment.[2] PSA has low specificity, and even when cancer is present, a single, screening PSA CANNOT distinguish between indolent and aggressive cancers.

The US Preventative Services Task Force (USPSTF) and the American Urological Association (AUA) have released the most complete evidence-based guidelines on using PSA for prostate cancer screening.[2,5] The primary points of the USPSTF guideline are summarized in **Box 1**, and those of the AUA guideline are summarized in **Box 2**. A comparison of the recommendations is shown in **Table 1**.

Box 1
US Preventative Services Task Force recommendations

"C" Recommendation[a]: Men aged 55 to 69 should make an individual decision about whether to be screened for prostate cancer with PSA, after a conversation with their doctor about the potential benefits and harms.

"D" Recommendation[b]: Men 70 years and older should not be screened for prostate cancer with PSA, even if they have higher risk for prostate cancer—the harms likely outweigh the benefits.

Men 55 to 69 with higher prostate cancer risk, such as men with a family history of metastatic prostate cancer and African American men, should also make an individual decision about screening after discussion with their doctor—there is not enough evidence on the high-risk groups to make a specific recommendation.

Men less than 55 should not be routinely screened, but may choose screening after a discussion with their doctor. There is very little information on the benefits and harms in this age group, although prostate cancer is much less common in these younger men.

Benefits of screening for prostate cancer include reduction in prostate cancer deaths by 0.1%, and reduction in metastatic prostate cancer by 0.3%, under optimal conditions in men aged 55 to 69.

Harms of screening include unnecessary biopsies, overdiagnosis of prostate cancer, and harms of active treatment, such as urinary incontinence and sexual dysfunction.

[a] C Recommendation: Some men may benefit from screening, but the balance of benefits and harms do not support routine screening.

[b] D Recommendation: Routine screening not recommended.

Data from Fenton JJ, Weyrich MS, Durbin S, et al. Prostate-specific antigen-based screening for prostate cancer: a systematic evidence review for the US Preventive Services Task Force. Evidence Synthesis No. 154. AHRQ Publication No. 17-05229-EF-1. Rockville (MD): Agency for Healthcare Research and Quality; 2018.

Box 2
American Urological Association recommendations on screening for prostate cancer

1. Men less than age 40 years: 1. The panel recommends against PSA screening in men less than 40 years (Recommendation; Evidence Strength Grade C)
2. Men aged 40 to 54 years: The panel does not recommend routine screening in men between ages 40 and 54 years at average risk (Recommendation; Evidence Strength Grade C)
3. [a] Men aged 55 to 69 years: The panel strongly recommends shared decision making for men who are considering PSA screening and proceeding based on a man's values and preferences (Standard; Evidence Strength Grade B)
4. To reduce the harms of screening, a routine screening interval of 2 years or more may be preferred over annual screening in those men who have participated in shared decision making and decided on screening. As compared with annual screening, it is expected that screening intervals of 2 years preserve most of the benefits and reduce overdiagnosis and false positives (Option; Evidence Strength Grade C)
5. Men age 70+ years: The panel does not recommend routine PSA screening in men age 70+ years or any man with less than a 10- to 15-year life expectancy (Recommendation; Evidence Strength Grade C)

[a] The greatest benefit of screening appears to be in men aged 55 to 69 years. Multiple approaches after a PSA test (eg, urinary and serum biomarkers, imaging, risk calculators) are available for identifying men more likely to harbor a prostate cancer and/or one with an aggressive phenotype. The use of such tools can be considered in men with a suspicious PSA level to inform prostate biopsy decisions.

[b] Grading the strength of evidence by the panel on the above guidelines was based on the quality of evidence as A (high), B (moderate), C (low). Standard was supported by evidence of higher quality (A, B), as compared with a recommendation (C).

From American Urological Association. Early detection of prostate cancer. Available at: https://www.auanet.org/guidelines/prostate-cancer-early-detection-(2013-reviewed-for-currency-2018). Accessed August 6, 2018; with permission.

Table 1
Comparison of US Preventative Services Task Force and American Urological Association guidelines on screening average risk asymptomatic men for early detection of prostate cancer

Age Group	USPSTF	AUA
<40	No routine screening, minimal evidence	Recommends against screening
40–54	No routine screening, minimal evidence	No routine screening; may choose screening after discussion with doctor
55–69	Shared decision making (C Recommendation)[a]	Shared decision making, strong recommendation (Standard)
>70 or life expectancy	Does not recommend	Does not recommend routinely
<10–15 y of life expectancy	Does not recommend	Does not recommend
Screening intervals	Periodic	Every 2–4 y

[a] C Recommendation: Some men may benefit from screening, but the balance of benefits and harms does not support routine screening.

Data from Fenton JJ, Weyrich MS, Durbin S, et al. Prostate-specific antigen-based screening for prostate cancer: a systematic evidence review for the US Preventive Services Task Force. Evidence Synthesis No. 154. AHRQ Publication No. 17-05229-EF-1. Rockville (MD): Agency for Healthcare Research and Quality; 2018; and American Urological Association. Early detection of prostate cancer. Available at: https://www.auanet.org/guidelines/prostate-cancer-early-detection-(2013-reviewed-for-currency-2018). Accessed August 6, 2018.

As **Boxes 1** and **2** and **Table 1** demonstrate, there is more agreement than disagreement between the 2 guidelines. Both guidelines recommend shared decision making for men aged 55 to 69, the "core group" for benefit from PSA screening.[2,5] Both guidelines do not recommend routine screening in men older or younger than men in the core group. Although the AUA calls shared decision making for the core group a standard based on grade B evidence, the USPSTF does not. The AUA also recommends shared decision making to guide possible screening in healthy men older than 69, whereas the USPSTF recommends against screening in that group.[2,5]

It is in the details of the screening offered that there is more uncertainty. The study site, which shows the most benefit of PSA screening, the ERSPC Swedish site in Goteborg, used the lowest PSA cutoff, 2.5 ng/dL, and a screening interval of every 2 years. However, the ERSPC overall allowed each site to set their own PSA cutoff values and intervals: cutoffs included 2.5 at the Swedish site, 3.0 at most sites, 4.0 at a few sites, and 10.0 initially at the Belgian site. The screening interval was every 4 years at most sites, but every 2 years at the Swedish site.[3] Interestingly, if a PSA obtained on a man in his 40s or 50s is less than the median for his age, the risk for prostate cancer 30 years in the future is lower. Similarly, if the PSA is less than 1 ng/mL, rescreening every 4 years is unlikely to miss a curable prostate cancer.[6]

The evidence for or against prostate cancer screening is mixed, and the studies are complicated by design flaws. However, it is unclear if better large prospective studies will be performed. Current evidence would be support the following conclusions:

1. Single PSA screening is likely of no benefit, unless the value is quite low for age. Neither the Stockholm Study, nor the much larger CAP Trial, showed benefit on prostate cancer mortality.[3,4]
2. Annual screening with PSA testing in men aged 50 to 69 years with a value of 4.0 ng/mL or more considered a positive result may be ineffective in reducing prostate cancer deaths. Although hampered by 78% of men in the control group undergoing PSA screening at least once during the study, the PLCO showed that there was no decrease in prostate cancer mortality nor in all-cause mortality. Furthermore, a PSA cutoff of 4.0 ng/mL was used in the prior US guidelines for prostate cancer screening to offer prostate biopsy. Such a practice likely resulted in overtreatment with most men (90%) in the PLCO who were diagnosed with prostate cancer choosing active treatment of the cancer with surgery, radiation, and/or hormonal therapy. This reflects the usual US practice.[2,3]

The ERSPC also suggests that a PSA cutoff of 4.0 ng/mL is not useful in reducing prostate cancer mortality. As noted above, PSA cutoffs varied from 2.5 ng/dL to 10.0 ng/dL in the different study centers, but most used a cutoff of 3.0 ng/mL by the end of the study. The centers using the lower PSA cutoffs accounted for the observed benefit of screening.[2]

3. Guidelines for PSA screening in the ERSPC are likely effective in reducing both metastatic prostate cancer and prostate cancer deaths, but at a substantial cost: increased biopsies, overdiagnosis, and overtreatment. The ERSPC showed an increased incidence of prostate cancer (RR 1.57) and reduced prostate cancer mortality with PSA screening for all men enrolled in the study. The center in Goteborg, Sweden demonstrated the most robust findings of reduction in prostate cancer mortality (RR, 0.58 [95% confidence interval [CI], 0.46–0.72]), but also had the lowest PSA cutoff (2.5 ng/dL) and the shortest screening interval (every 2 years, vs every 4 years at most centers).[2]

Four ERSPC centers (Sweden, the Netherlands, Finland, and Switzerland) assessed the cumulative incidence of metastatic prostate cancer. Among these centers, Sweden and the Netherlands showed a significant reduction in prostate cancer mortality, but the other 2 did not. At 12 years' follow-up, metastatic prostate cancer was reduced (RR, 0.70 [95% CI, 0.60–0.82]; *P* = .001).[2]

However, these benefits come at significant cost: the 4 centers compiling data on metastatic cancer showed a 55.6% increased incidence of prostate cancer in the intervention arms. Twelve men, many of whom may have had indolent cancers, needed to be diagnosed with prostate cancer to avert one case of metastatic cancer. In the ERSPC as a whole, there were 32.3 positive screens and 27.7 biopsies per 100 men randomized to screening, yet 75.8% of the biopsies were negative for cancer.[2] More aggressive treatments, especially radical prostatectomy, are most likely to prevent metastatic prostate cancer and prostate cancer deaths, yet this surgery also doubles the risk of both erectile dysfunction and urinary incontinence.[1]

4. There is almost no information on the value of PSA screening for high-risk groups. The PLCO Trial did not include enough African American men, nor men with a positive family history, to separately assess the effect of PSA screening. However, in the overall PLCO Trial, 4833 men had a positive family history, and the trend for prostate cancer deaths favored screening (RR 0.49 [95% CI, 0.22–1.10]; *P* = .08).[2] Only one site in the ERSPC asked about family history, and that only in the intervention arm, so relative benefit of screening could not be assessed; the number of men in the control arm with a positive family history was unknown.[2]
5. Harms occur on multiple levels with PSA screening. Psychological harms of false-positive PSA screens have been minimally studied, but are likely more than trivial. Harms of prostate core biopsy are better documented: at the ERSPC Rotterdam site, 22.6% had hematuria greater than 3 days; 7.5% had significant postoperative pain; 3.5% had fever; and 0.5% were hospitalized, mostly for infections. Hematospermia as well as urinary and infectious complications was more prevalent in other studies of biopsy sequelae. All active treatments, not just radical prostatectomy, carry high rates of erectile dysfunction, urinary incontinence, and bowel problems. Finally, overdiagnosis, the identification of indolent prostate cancers, is a major source of harm: the USPSTF calculated that 16.4% of the prostate cancers identified in the PLCO Trial, and 33.2% of those identified in the ERSPC Trial, were overdiagnosed. Given the US rate of 90% active treatments, overdiagnosis represents both a huge expense without benefit and a source of posttreatment harms, also without benefit.[2]

SUMMARY

Based on current evidence, prostate cancer screening by any method other than PSA is not supported. Screening men younger than 55 or older than 70 routinely is not supported. PSA screening in men 55 to 69 is most likely to reduce prostate metastasis and death if a lower PSA cutoff is used (2.5 or 3.0 ng/mL), and men are willing to undergo biopsy and active treatment at higher rates than are being performed now. However, active surveillance for less-risky cancers must increase, to lower rates of overdiagnosis and overtreatment. For these reasons, the decision should be made individually between doctor and patient, after discussion.

REFERENCES

1. DynaMed. Accessed March 18, 2018.

2. Fenton JJ, Weyrich MS, Durbin S, et al. Prostate-specific antigen-based screening for prostate cancer: a systematic evidence review for the U.S. preventive services task force. Rockville (MD): Agency for Healthcare Research and Quality; 2018. Evidence Synthesis No. 154. AHRQ Publication No. 17-05229-EF-1.
3. Lin K, Croswell JM, Koenig H, et al. Prostate-specific antigen-based screening for prostate cancer: an evidence update for the U.S. preventive services task force. Rockville (MD): Agency for Healthcare Research and Quality; 2011. Evidence Synthesis No. 90. AHRQ Publication No. 12-05160-EF-1.
4. Martin RM, Donovan JL, Turner EL, et al. Efeect of a low-intensity PSA-based screening intervention on prostate cancer mortality: the CAP randomized clinical trial. JAMA 2018;319(9):883–95.
5. American Urological Association. Early detection of prostate cancer. Available at: http://www.auanet.org/guidelines/prostate-cancer-early-detection-(2013-reviewed-for-currency-2018. Accessed August 6, 2018.
6. Carter HB. American Urological Association (AUA) guidelines on prostate cancer detection process and rationale. BJU Int 2013;112(5):543–7.

Hematuria

Leah M. Peterson, MD[a,*], Henry S. Reed, MD[b]

KEYWORDS

- Hematuria • Gross hematuria • Microscopic hematuria • Cystoscopy
- CT urography • Urine cytology

KEY POINTS

- There is insufficient evidence to recommend screening urinalysis for the detection of bladder cancer in the absence of clinical indicators.
- More than 10% of patients with gross hematuria have an underlying malignancy. Any patient with gross hematuria should be referred for urologic evaluation.
- Urine cytology is not recommended as part of the initial work-up of hematuria.
- Clinicians should pursue evaluation of hematuria even if the patient is receiving antiplatelet or anticoagulant therapy.

BACKGROUND

Hematuria is defined as the presence of red blood cells in the urine, and is a problem commonly encountered by primary care physicians. At present, screening healthy, asymptomatic patients with urinalysis for the purpose of cancer detection is not recommended by any major health organization. The US Preventive Services Task Force (USPSTF) has issued an "I" recommendation because of insufficient evidence on the benefits and harms of screening, and the American Urological Association (AUA) does not recommend routine screening of asymptomatic individuals. Thus, microscopic hematuria is typically found incidentally in a urinalysis ordered for another indication.

Hematuria is further categorized into gross hematuria and microscopic hematuria. Gross hematuria is sufficient to be evident to the naked eye of the patient or examiner (>50 red blood cells [RBCs] per high-power field [HPF]), whereas microscopic hematuria is not evident without microscopic analysis of the urine sample. Microscopic hematuria is defined as greater than or equal to 3 RBCs per HPF on a properly collected urine sample. Although these two differ in quantification, there is substantial overlap in the underlying differential diagnoses for both. The differential diagnoses for both gross and microscopic hematuria are extensive, as noted in **Box 1**. Furthermore, finding one

Disclosure: The authors have nothing to disclose.
[a] Smoky Hill Family Medicine Residency Program, Salina, KS, USA; [b] Internal Medicine/Nephrology, Mowery Clinic, 737 East Crawford, Salina, KS 67401, USA
* Corresponding author. 651 East Prescott, Salina, KS 67401.
E-mail address: lpeterson@salinahealth.org

Prim Care Clin Office Pract 46 (2019) 265–273
https://doi.org/10.1016/j.pop.2019.02.008

Box 1
Differential diagnosis of hematuria

Malignancy
- Renal
- Bladder
- Prostate

Benign tumors (endometriosis of the urinary tract)

Infection
- Urethritis
- Cystitis
- Viral illness
- Upper urinary tract infection
- Endocarditis
- Visceral abscesses
- Schistosomiasis
- Tuberculosis
- Syphilis

Menstruation

Urolithiasis

Trauma
- Exercise induced (resolves with rest)
- Abdominal trauma or pelvic fracture with injury to urinary tract
- Iatrogenic (abdominal or pelvic surgery, chronic indwelling catheter)
- Foreign body (physical/sexual abuse)

Congenital/familial
- Cystic disease (polycystic kidney disease, solitary cyst)
- Alport syndrome
- Fabry disease
- Renal tubular acidosis type 1

Urinary anatomic
- Urethral stricture
- Posterior urethral valve
- Hydronephrosis
- Benign prostatic hyperplasia

Chemical
- Aminoglycosides
- Cyclosporine
- Oral contraceptives
- Chinese herbs

Hematologic/vascular
- Bleeding dyscrasia (hemophilia)
- Sickle cell anemia/trait
- Hemangioma
- Arteriovenous malformation (rare)
- Renal artery/vein thrombosis
- Arterial emboli to kidney

Renal disease
- Radiation nephritis and cystitis
- Tubulointerstitial nephritis (caused by drugs, infections, systemic disease)
- Membranoproliferative, poststreptococcal, or rapidly progressive glomerulonephritis
- Immunoglobulin A nephropathy
- Lupus nephritis
- Henoch-Schönlein purpura
- Goodpasture syndrome

evident cause for hematuria does not necessarily exclude other potentially dangerous causes.

Among the potential causes for this problem, occult malignancy is of most concern.[1] From 10% to 40% of individuals with a single episode of gross hematuria have an underlying malignancy.[2] Microscopic hematuria more commonly has benign causes. Common benign causes include menstruation, vigorous exercise, viral illness, recent urinary tract procedure, trauma, urinary tract infection, benign prostatic hyperplasia, and urinary calculi.[3] However, up to 5% of patients with asymptomatic microscopic hematuria have an underlying malignancy.[2]

Because of the concern for occult malignancy in patient with hematurias, assessment for risk factors for malignancy and longitudinal follow-up is essential. Patient age, gender, and presence of risk factors can aid primary care physicians in narrowing the differential and determining the appropriate diagnostic and management plan. Men, people more than 35 years of age, and people with more than a 10-pack-year smoking history have an increased risk of malignancy. In 2012, the AUA published updated guidelines for the diagnosis, evaluation, and management of asymptomatic microscopic hematuria in adults. That guideline details the current recommended approach for management of patients with hematuria in the primary care setting, and serves as the basis for the information in this article.

EPIDEMIOLOGY

Hematuria is a common finding in clinical practice. Prevalence rates for microscopic hematuria vary from 1% to 18%, depending on patient age, gender, frequency of testing, and presence of risk factors.[3] In many patients with hematuria, a specific cause or disorder is not found. Nevertheless, adhering to AUA guidelines for evaluation is critical, given the potential for occult malignancy described earlier. The cancer yield in the work-up of hematuria exceeds that for screening colonoscopy by 10-fold, but referral rates for hematuria in high-risk patients have been found to be as low as 12.8%.[4]

Risk factors for malignancy are numerous, and are noted in **Table 1**. Bladder cancer is the fourth most common cancer occurring in the United States. Cigarette smoking is the number 1 environmental risk factor associated with the development of urologic malignancy, specifically urothelial carcinoma. Smoking is known to increase people's risk of bladder cancer by at least 3-fold, and is associated with 50% to 66% of bladder cancers in men and 25% of bladder cancers in women.[5] Work-related contact with cyclic chemicals, such as benzene dyes, accounts for an additional 25% of bladder cancers.[5] Persons with professions involving heavy exposure to dyes, rubbers, textiles, paints, leathers, and chemicals show an increased risk of bladder cancer, and clinicians should maintain an increased index of suspicion in these cases.[5]

It should be noted that the recommendations for management of hematuria are based on expert opinion and low-quality evidence, because the evidence is limited to mainly observational studies with small sample sizes, done with heterogeneous study designs on variable populations.

The differential diagnosis for hematuria is extensive, as noted in **Table 1**.

WORK-UP AND TREATMENT

Gross Hematuria

Gross hematuria may be symptomatic or asymptomatic, but it is usually brought to the clinician's attention by the patient. Gross hematuria is less common than microscopic

Table 1
Risk factors for malignancy in patients with hematuria

Male gender	—
Age>50 y	—
Current smoker	—
History of smoking	—
Occupational exposure	—
Aromatic amines	Chimney sweeps, nurses, waiters, tire manufacturers; and Aluminum, ship, and oil/petroleum workers
Polycyclic aromatic hydrocarbons	Tobacco, dye, rubber, and leather workers; hairdressers; and printers
Aminobiphenyl	—
Arsenic	—
Analgesic abuse	Phenacetin
History of gross hematuria	—
Chronic urinary tract infection	*Schistosoma haematobium*
Chronic indwelling foreign body	Foley catheter
History of urologic disorder or disease	—
History of irritative voiding symptoms	—
Cancer treatments	Cyclophosphamide, ifosfamide, pelvic radiation
Chinese herbs	Aristolochic

hematuria but more often has a dangerous cause. As previously stated, pretest probability for malignancy is high for gross hematuria. The presence of pain in a patient with hematuria can narrow the list of potential diagnoses. Symptomatic gross hematuria with associated flank pain or renal colic is the classic presentation of urinary stone disease, but painless gross hematuria is more strongly associated with an underlying malignancy.[6]

Primary care physicians should maintain a low threshold for urology consultation in the setting of gross hematuria. If a benign cause is not immediately evident, prompt urologic referral is needed, because rates of malignancy in gross hematuria are 10% to 40%. However, even in patients with an identifiable cause, urology consultation is still recommended, because of the high prevalence of dangerous causes for gross hematuria, especially in patients with risk factors for malignancy.[6] For these reasons, the author recommends prompt urologic consultation in all patients with gross hematuria.

In addition to urologic referral, patients who present with gross hematuria should have a thorough investigation for signs of intrinsic renal damage. Urine microscopy is recommended to assess for red cell casts. In addition to urinalysis with microscopy, assessing renal function and albumin levels is recommended. Quantification of urine protein is also recommended, either through 24-hour urine sampling or with a spot urine microalbumin/creatinine ratio. A reading of greater than 300 mg protein daily (or equivalent ratio) is considered diagnostic for proteinuria.

Urologic work-up for the evaluation of gross hematuria often includes cystoscopy. Cystoscopy is indicated for patients who are 35 years of age and older or have risk factors for malignancy.[3] Cystoscopy allows direct visualization of the bladder and can detect malignancy or other sources of bleeding. It should be noted that cystoscopy is preferred to urine cytology in the work-up of hematuria, because of its improved sensitivity compared with urine cytology.[7]

The overall approach to diagnostic management for gross hematuria is noted in **Fig. 1**.

Microscopic Hematuria

Microscopic hematuria is defined as the presence of 3 RBCs per HPF on microscopic analysis of a properly collected and analyzed urine sample, with no obvious benign cause.[3] The use of a simple urine dipstick test in identification of hematuria has a high false-positive rate, necessitating use of follow-up microscopic evaluation of all positive dipstick results. The presence of hemoglobinuria, myoglobinuria, semen, highly alkaline urine (pH>9), and concentrated urine can cause a false-positive result for blood on dipstick analysis.[7] Further, vitamin C has been shown to cause false-negative results on dipstick testing, because of the reducing properties of vitamin C.[8]

Microscopic examination of the urine is the most important test in the evaluation of hematuria.[3] Proper collection and analysis of the urine sample is as follows. At least 10 mL of urine should be collected via a midstream catch and should be immediately centrifuged at 2000 revolutions per minute for 10 minutes. The supernatant should then be discarded and the sediment suspended in 0.3 mL of supernatant and/or saline. Next, at least 10 to 20 microscopic fields should be examined under 400× magnification.[7] If the specimen shows large amounts of squamous epithelial cells (more than 5 per HPF), or if the patient is unable to provide an uncontaminated specimen secondary to anatomic constraints (eg, obesity or phimosis), catheterization should be used to obtain a specimen.[3]

Patients in whom dipstick testing is positive but subsequent microscopic evaluation is negative should undergo 3 additional microscopic tests to rule out microscopic hematuria. This recommendation is based on expert opinion, and the timing of repeat

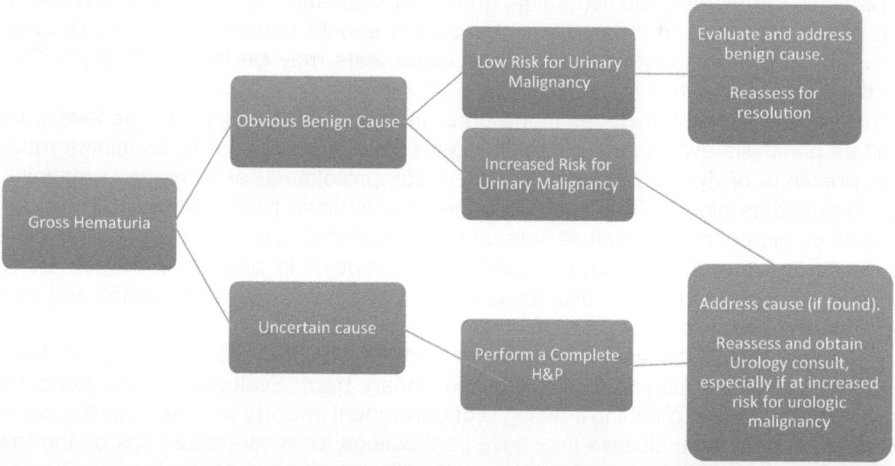

Fig. 1. Approach to gross hematuria. Maintain low threshold for urology consultation. Obtain concurrent nephrology consultation if signs of glomerular disease are present. H&P, history and physical.

testing is not defined by the AUA guidelines. The authors recommend repeat testing every 4 to 6 weeks for 3 additional tests. If one of the subsequent tests is positive for hematuria on microscopy, the patient is considered to have a diagnosis of microscopic hematuria and should be managed as per AUA guidelines outlined in this article. If all 3 subsequent samples are negative on microscopy, the patient does not require further evaluation for hematuria, but other causes for positive dipstick result, namely hemoglobinuria and myoglobinuria, should be considered.

If microscopic hematuria is detected in the presence of pyuria, a urine culture should be obtained to rule out urinary tract infection. If infection is present, it should be treated appropriately and a microscopic urinalysis should be repeated in 6 weeks to assess for resolution of hematuria.[3] If the hematuria has resolved, no further work-up is required. If microscopic hematuria is noted to be persistent, further work-up is recommended.

It should be noted that the presence of microscopic hematuria should not be solely ascribed to the use of anticoagulant medications. Although use of these medications can exacerbate any bleeding that is present, they should not be attributed as the sole cause of hematuria. Asymptomatic microscopic hematuria in patients who are taking anticoagulants requires urologic and nephrologic evaluation, regardless of the type of anticoagulant therapy.[9] The work-up in these patients is identical to that of patients not taking anticoagulant medications.

On detection of microscopic hematuria, clinicians should perform a complete history and physical examination, including measurement of blood pressure and laboratory assessment. The history and physical can help rule out benign causes of microscopic hematuria and reveal potential causes and risk factors for malignancy. A pelvic examination should be performed in women to identify urethral masses, diverticula, atrophic vaginitis, or a uterine source of bleeding.[7] A rectal examination is necessary in men to evaluate the size and presence of nodularity in the prostate.[7]

A single urinalysis with hematuria is common and often has a benign cause. Benign causes of microscopic hematuria include infection, menstruation, vigorous exercise, medical renal disease, viral illness, trauma, or recent urologic procedure (eg, Foley catheterization). If a benign cause is identified, it should be treated and a repeat evaluation for microscopic hematuria should be performed 6 weeks later. If this repeat test is negative for microscopic hematuria, no further evaluation is necessary. However, if the microscopic hematuria persists, the patient should undergo further evaluation. Renal function should be evaluated, and other tests may be indicated, depending on the pertinent findings in the history and physical.

The renal evaluation includes blood urea nitrogen (BUN) and creatinine levels, as well as urinalysis evaluation for protein and a spot urine protein to creatinine ratio. The presence of dysmorphic RBCs, RBC casts, proteinuria, or increased creatinine levels suggests glomerular injury and underlying intrinsic renal disease. Glomerular causes of microscopic hematuria warrant prompt referral to a nephrology subspecialist for further investigation and possible renal biopsy.[7] In patients with glomerular bleeding, the most common diagnoses are immunoglobulin A nephropathy and thin basement membrane nephropathy.[7]

If intrinsic renal disease is noted, the patient should receive evaluation from nephrology before imaging to evaluate the urinary tract. Evaluation of the patient's renal function before pursuing imaging is of paramount importance, because the presence of intrinsic renal disease may have implications for renal-related risk during the evaluation and management of patients with microscopic hematuria.[3]

After testing for renal disease is completed, imaging of the upper urinary tract is the next step. This imaging can be performed by the primary care provider, before urologic consultation.[10] Historically, intravenous pyelography was the preferred choice for upper tract imaging, but intravenous pyelography has largely been replaced by computed tomography (CT) urography. CT urography combines a noncontrast phase to diagnose hydronephrosis and urinary calculi, a nephrogenic phase to evaluate the renal parenchyma for pyelonephritis or neoplastic lesions, and an excretory phase to detect urothelial disease.[7] In one prospective study that compared CT urography and intravenous pyelography in the same patients with microscopic hematuria, sensitivity and accuracy of CT were 100% and 98.3% compared with 60.5% and 80.9% for intravenous pyelography.[11] Because the risk of missed diagnoses with intravenous pyelography is significant, and it tends to require additional imaging on a more frequent basis, CT urography is preferred.[10]

One concern with CT urography is radiation exposure. The average radiation dose with CT urography (7 mSv) is more than double that of intravenous pyelography (3 mSv).[12] New lower-dose protocols and synchronous acquisition of nephrogenic and excretory phase images are now used in an attempt to decrease radiation exposure. These split-bolus CT urography protocols provide equivalent if not superior visualization of the upper urinary tracts, reduced radiation exposure, and added logistic convenience.[13]

CT urography is not recommended in radiation-sensitive populations (eg, pregnant women) and in persons with renal insufficiency or allergy to contrast media.[7] In these situations, alternative imaging should be obtained. Magnetic resonance urography (without/with intravenous contrast) is the recommended imaging modality in these patients, because it provides high diagnostic sensitivity and specificity in imaging of the renal parenchyma.[3] Magnetic resonance urography is notably more expensive than CT urography, and is inferior at detecting stone disease, a common cause for hematuria. Further, the role of magnetic resonance urography in visualizing the collecting system is indeterminate. Thus, in patients with contraindications to CT in whom collecting system detail is deemed imperative, combining magnetic resonance urography with retrograde pyelogram is recommended.[3]

If the patient has contraindications to MRI (eg, presence of metal in the body) as well as contraindications to contrast CT, noncontrast CT with retrograde pyelogram or renal ultrasonography with retrograde pyelogram provides alternative evaluation.[3] This approach is also recommended in moderate to severe renal disease, because these patients are now advised to avoid gadolinium-enhanced MRI because of risk of nephrogenic systemic fibrosis.[14]

Renal ultrasonography alone is less sensitive in detecting urothelial and renal masses, and does not produce diagnostic certainty. Use of renal ultrasonography in the setting of hematuria may lead to indeterminate findings that necessitate additional imaging and costs.[7] There are emerging data to support the use of ultrasonography with cystoscopy as an alternative diagnostic approach to the use of CT urography, but further research is needed to support a practice change.[1]

Pregnant women with hematuria require special consideration. Malignancies in this low-risk group (typically <40 years of age), are rare. The AUA guidelines recommend magnetic resonance urography, MRI with retrograde pyelogram, or ultrasonography to screen for major renal lesions, with a full work-up to be performed after delivery, if needed. This full postpartum work-up is only to be performed if hematuria persists after gynecologic bleeding and persistent infection have been ruled out.[3] Most cases of microscopic hematuria in pregnant women are caused by non–life-threatening conditions, and occult malignancy is identified in fewer than 5% of cases.[3]

On completion of one of the imaging strategies discussed earlier, the next step in the evaluation of microscopic hematuria is cystoscopy. Cystoscopy is recommended in all patients with asymptomatic microscopic hematuria who present with risk factors for malignancy (see **Box 1**), regardless of age. Cystoscopy enables diagnosis of

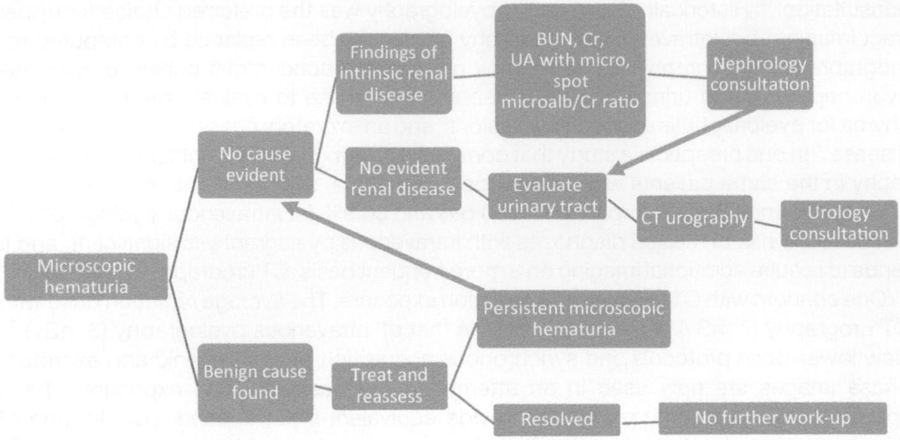

Fig. 2. Asymptomatic hematuria. Cr, creatinine; micro, microscopy; microalb, microalbumin; UA, urinalysis. (*Data from* Davis R, Jones JS, Barocas DA, et al. Diagnosis, evaluation and follow-up of asymptomatic microscopic hematuria (AMH) in adults: AUA guideline. J Urol 2012;188:2473–81.)

urethral strictures, benign prostatic hyperplasia, and bladder masses through direct visualization of the lower urinary tract. In patients younger than 35 years, cystoscopy is performed only at the discretion of a urologist, because the likelihood of urinary tract malignancy is low.[3]

As previously stated, cytology is no longer recommended as a routine part of the evaluation of microscopic hematuria. There are still some indications for urine cytology, particularly in patients with risk factors for carcinoma in situ (irritative voiding symptoms, tobacco use, chemical exposures).[3] However, given the superior sensitivity of cystoscopy in diagnosis, and the issues with interpretation subjectivity in urine cytology, cystoscopy is preferred in most cases. Further, the new rapid urinary assays or bladder cancer detection may be preferred by some specialists. These tests do not currently have evidence showing superiority to cystoscopy or cytology in the initial detection of urothelial malignancies,[15] and the author recommends that these tests not be ordered by primary care physicians.

If the appropriate work-up is completed and does not reveal nephrologic or urologic disease, the patient should have urinalysis with microscopy performed on an annual basis for at least 2 years. If these two repeat tests do not reveal persistence of the hematuria, the risk of future malignancy is less than 1%.[16,17] In this situation, no further surveillance is necessary. However, if the asymptomatic microscopic hematuria persists over this time, the patient should have a full repeat evaluation 3 to 5 years after the initial work-up.[3] It should be noted that patient-specific risk factors for malignancy can help guide clinical decision making regarding the timing of repeat work-up.[17]

The diagnostic work-up for asymptomatic microscopic hematuria is summarized in **Fig. 2**.

REFERENCES

1. Halpern JA, Chughtai B, Ghomrawi H. Cost-effectiveness of common diagnostic approaches for evaluation of asymptomatic microscopic hematuria. JAMA Intern Med 2017;6:800–6.

2. Khadra MH, Pickard RS, Charlton M, et al. A prospective analysis of 1,930 patients with hematuria to evaluate current diagnostic practice. J Urol 2000;163: 524–7.
3. Davis R, Jones JS, Barocas DA, et al. Diagnosis, evaluation and follow-up of asymptomatic microscopic hematuria (AMH) in adults: AUA guideline. J Urol 2012;188:2473–81.
4. Elias K, Svatek RS, Gupta S, et al. High risk patients with hematuria are not evaluated according to guideline recommendations. Cancer 2010;12:2954–9.
5. Pashos CL, Botteman MF, Laskin BL, et al. Bladder cancer: epidemiology, diagnosis, and management. Cancer Pract 2002;6:311–22.
6. Nielsen M, Qaseem A. Hematuria as a marker of occult urinary tract cancer: advice for high-value care from the American college of physicians. Ann Intern Med 2016;164:488–97.
7. Sharp VJ, Barnes KT, Erickson BA. Assessment of asymptomatic microscopic hematuria in adults. Am Fam Physician 2013;11:748–54.
8. Brigden ML, Edgell D, McPherson M, et al. High incidence of significant urinary ascorbic acid concentrations in a west coast population—implications for routine urinalysis. Clin Chem 1992;3:426–31.
9. Van Savage JG, Fried FA. Anticoagulant associated hematuria: a prospective study. J Urol 1995;5:1594–6.
10. Ramchandani P, Kisler T, Francis IR, et al. Expert panel on urologic imaging. ACR appropriateness criteria: hematuria. Reston (VA): American College of Radiology; 2014. Available at: https://acsearch.acr.org/docs/69490/Narrative/. Accessed July 19, 2018.
11. Gray Sears CL, Ward JF, Sears ST, et al. Prospective comparison of computerized tomography and excretory urography in the initial evaluation of asymptomatic microhematuria. J Urol 2002;168(6):2457–60.
12. Eikefjord EN, Thorsen F, Rorvik J. Comparison of effective radiation doses in patients undergoing unenhanced MDCT and excretory urography for acute flank pain. AJR Am J Roentgenol 2007;4:934–9.
13. Chow LC, Kwan SW, Olcott EW, et al. Split-bolus MDCT urography with synchronous nephrographic and excretory phase enhancement. AJR Am J Roentgenol 2007;2:314–22.
14. Wiginton CD, Kelly B, Oto A, et al. Gadolinium-based contrast exposure, nephrogenic systemic fibrosis, and gadolinium detection in tissue. AJR Am J Roentgenol 2008;4:1060–8.
15. Glas AS, Roos D, Deutekom M, et al. Tumor markers in the diagnosis of primary bladder cancer. A systematic review. J Urol 2003;6:1975–82.
16. Madeb R, Golijanin D, Knopf J, et al. Long-term outcome of patients with a negative work-up for asymptomatic microhematuria. Urology 2010;1:20–5.
17. Edwards TJ, Dickinson AJ, Gosling J, et al. Patient-specific risk of undetected malignant disease after investigation for haematuria, based on a 4-year follow-up. BJU Int 2011;2:247–52.

Urologic Malignancies

Jennifer E. Thuener, MD

KEYWORDS

• Renal cell carcinoma • Kidney cancer • Bladder cancer • Incidental renal mass

KEY POINTS

- Bladder cancer can be identified by hematuria, and is more easily treated when identified early. Primary care doctors should be familiar with symptoms and management.
- Renal cancer is generally asymptomatic, however primary care physicians should be familiar with risk factors and be knowledgeable of the workup of incidental renal masses.

OVERVIEW

Cancer remained the second leading cause of death in the United States in 2014 and plays a significant role in morbidity and mortality of patients.[1] Cancer was the leading cause of death in both men and women ages 60 to 79, with 22% of all deaths in 2015 attributed to cancer.[1] Bladder and kidney cancer are projected to account for 150,350 new cases of urologic malignancy in 2018. Most urologic malignancies occur in men, with bladder cancer being the most common urologic malignancy in men and the fourth most common cancer diagnosis overall. In 2018, 7% of all new cancer diagnoses and 4% of cancer deaths in men are attributable to bladder cancer.[1] Bladder cancer is much less common in women, but does still occur.

Primary care physicians play a key role in the early diagnosis and early referral for definitive management of both bladder and kidney cancer. Given that both renal and bladder cancer have improved 5-year survival rates when diagnosed as a localized tumor,[1] it is vital that primary care physicians are aware of concerning symptoms and signs of bladder and kidney cancer that need to be further evaluated.

BLADDER CANCER

Bladder cancer is an overarching term that describes a number of tumors that arise from the urothelial lining of the bladder, renal pelvis, ureters, and urethra.[2] Most bladder cancers in the United States are located in the bladder, although there are a small number of cancers that are found in the ureters, urethra, and renal pelvis. Most tumors are urothelial carcinomas.[2,3]

Disclosure Statement: The author has nothing to disclose.
Department of Family and Community Medicine, University of Kansas Medical Center, 850 North Hillside, Wichita, KS 67226, USA
E-mail address: jthuener@kumc.edu

Prim Care Clin Office Pract 46 (2019) 275–285
https://doi.org/10.1016/j.pop.2019.02.009 primarycare.theclinics.com
0095-4543/19/

When diagnosed as carcinoma in situ, 96% of patients with bladder cancer will survive for 5 years. However, only 51% of bladder cancer is diagnosed at this early stage.[1] The 5-year survival rate of bladder cancer diagnosed in all stages is 77%. Although 51% of bladder cancer is diagnosed in situ, 34% is diagnosed in a localized stage, 7% regional and 4% distant.[1]

Bladder cancer can present as a spectrum of disease from a low-grade papillary lesion to an invasive, infiltrative disease process. The bladder consists of 4 layers: (1) epithelial, (2) subepithelial connective tissue (lamina propria), (3) muscle (muscularis propria), and (4) perivesical fat. The details of staging are noted in. Bladder cancer management is divided into non–muscle invasive (Stages 0–1) and muscle invasive (stages 2–4).[2]

Muscle-invasive bladder cancer has high morbidity and mortality. Currently, there are no recommendations for routine screening for bladder cancer, thus the primary care physician should advise patients on risk modification and early detection and treatment.

Risk Factors

Both modifiable and nonmodifiable risk factors are well described for bladder cancer. Male sex is the most notable nonmodifiable risk factor, with bladder cancer occurring 3 times more often in men compared with women.[4] Although men have a higher incidence, women have a higher mortality when diagnosed. This increased mortality may be the result of women being diagnosed at a later stage.[5] In addition, slow acetylation of N-acetyltransferase 2, a genetically inherited risk factor, may increase susceptibility of cellular damage to carcinogens, such as tobacco smoke, increasing the likelihood of developing bladder cancer as a result of carcinogen exposure.[4–6]

Established modifiable risk factors for bladder cancer include tobacco smoke and exposure to occupational chemicals.[5] Tobacco smoking is estimated to contribute to 50% of bladder cancer diagnoses.[5] Tobacco smoke contains many carcinogens that are renally excreted, and the direct contact with the urinary system produces the increased risk of tumor. Historically, men have had a higher rate of smoking than women, which may account for higher rates of bladder cancer in men. Recent increases in the incidence of bladder cancer in women may be partially explained by smoking rates that have been similar in men and women the United States since the 1970s and a bladder cancer latency period of more than 30 years.[6]

Another key risk factor for bladder cancer is occupational exposure to aromatic amines, polycyclic aromatic hydrocarbons, and chlorinated hydrocarbons. These substances are found mainly in industrial areas processing paint, metal, and petroleum products. As industry is becoming more aware of these risks, the exposure of patients to these carcinogens has dropped.[5]

Coffee, alcohol, and amount of water intake have not been attributed to increasing risk. Similarly, a 2013 study confirmed that ingestion of red meat and obesity are also not risk factors.[5]

Screening

There is currently no recommended screening for bladder cancer in adults. The US Preventive Services Task Force has a recommendation of I, indicating that there is not sufficient current evidence to recommend for or against screening.[7]

Clinical Presentation

Gross or microscopic, painless hematuria is the most common presenting symptom for bladder cancer, with 85% of patients diagnosed with bladder cancer noting hematuria as a presenting complaint.[3] Although both microscopic and gross hematuria can raise clinical concern for bladder cancer, gross hematuria is far more concerning. Gross hematuria has a 3-year positive predictive value of bladder cancer of 7.4% in men, and 3.4% in women.[3] Microscopic hematuria is defined as more than 3 red blood cells (RBCs) per high power field during urine microscopy, whereas gross hematuria is urine that is noted to be pink, red, or brown with RBCs noted on urine microscopy. Urine color alone should not be used to confirm hematuria, as many things can cause changes in urine pigment, including phenazopyridine, vegetable dyes, beets, urates, free myoglobin, and infection with serratia marcescens. Hematuria may or may not be accompanied by irritative symptoms.

Diagnosis

If a primary care physician is concerned about bladder malignancy, referral to a urologist for further workup is recommended. Investigation of suspected bladder cancer generally includes a computed tomography (CT) urography or MRI to evaluate the upper urinary tract and a cystoscopy to evaluate the lower urinary tract.[4]

Cystoscopy allows direct visualization of the bladder to confirm the diagnosis with visualization of the tumor. Visible tumor or any areas of redness or inflammation are removed for pathologic staging in a procedure performed via cystoscopy, known as transurethral resection of bladder tumor (TURBT). It is recommended that there is a pelvic examination under anesthesia to clinically determine invasion, both before and after the TURBT procedure.[4] TURBT should be used on all identified lesions to assess for cancer depth and to determine staging of the tumor.[4] Tumor depth will place the tumor into the categories of non–muscle-invasive (NMIBC) or muscle-invasive bladder cancer (MIBC).

An abdominal ultrasound is not sufficient for ruling out tumors of the upper urinary tract.[4] At this time, urine cytology is not indicated for the initial workup of asymptomatic microscopic hematuria, as it has low sensitivity for all bladder cancer. However, urine cytology may be used in surveillance of some patients with bladder cancer.[8]

Management

For management and prognosis, bladder cancer is categorized into NMIBC and MIBC, as these 2 entities have different management and prognosis.

Non–muscle-invasive tumors accounted for 75% of all new bladder cancers in 2015.[4] These tumors can be noninvasive papillary tumors, carcinoma in situ, or tumors that are infiltrating only into the lamina propria. Non–muscle-invasive tumors are given a pathologic designation of low or high grade, which is used to determine management and prognosis.

The American Urologic Association (AUA) risk stratifies NMIBC to help determine optimal treatment strategies. The risk stratification system identifies the risk for progression of NMIBC and is based on size, number, type, and grade of lesions as well as recurrence. At each occurrence or recurrence of disease, the physician assigns the patient a risk level of low, intermediate, or high.[4]

Initial management of all NMIBC is full visualization and resection of all identified abnormal tissue. Further management is based on risk level identified by the lesions and pathology. Generally, patients with low-risk tumors are treated with a single instillation of intravesical chemotherapy within 24 hours of the TURBT and have no further treatment for that occurrence of disease. In intermediate-risk patients, treatment consists of instillation of intravesical chemotherapy at time of TURBT, as well as maintenance treatment with intravesical chemotherapy for 1 year.[3] For patients with high-risk NMIBC, intravesical immunotherapy with bacille Calmette-Guerin vaccine (BCG)

vaccination for 3 years. Treatment with immunotherapy has been shown to reduce recurrences and delay disease progression (**Table 1**).[3]

Muscle-invasive tumors account for the minority of bladder cancer, but have significantly higher mortality than non–muscle-invasive types.[8] While treatment of non–muscle-invasive disease focuses on bladder-sparing therapies, the mainstay in treatment of MIBC is radical cystectomy and bilateral pelvic lymphadenopathy, along with neoadjuvant chemotherapy. Twenty-five percent of patients with new bladder cancer will have muscle-invasive disease at time of diagnosis, and 50% of patients with high-risk NMIBC can progress to muscle-invasive disease.[8] During evaluation of MIBC, care should be taken to evaluate for metastatic disease, as this will change management. Risks of a radical cystectomy include short-term and long-term complications, such as incontinence and impaired sexual function. Due to the anatomic location of the bladder in relation to other pelvic organs, a radical cystectomy involves the removal of the bladder, prostate, and seminal vesicles in men and the bladder, uterus, fallopian tubes, ovaries, and anterior vaginal wall in women.[3,8] In addition to radical cystectomy, patients may be offered neoadjuvant chemotherapy if physically able to tolerate. The AUA recommends only using cisplatin-based neoadjuvant chemotherapy; however, toxicity may limit cisplatin use in up to 50% of patients.[8]

Patients found to have metastatic disease are treated with cisplatin-based chemotherapy or palliation only without surgical intervention. The median survival of patients with metastatic disease is 14 months.[9]

Follow-up/Surveillance

For patients with low-risk, NMIBC, cystoscopy should be repeated 3 months after TURBT. If negative at 3 months, cystoscopy should be repeated again at 1 year after diagnosis. If both cystoscopies show no recurrence or progression, annual cystoscopy for 5 years is recommended by the AUA. There is no need to do surveillance cytology or upper urinary tract imaging in low-risk patients.[10]

If the patient has intermediate-risk NMIBC, the physician should use clinical judgment to determine if the lesion seems more low or high risk. Consequently, treatment should follow the guidelines for low-risk or high-risk tumors depending on clinician judgment.[8]

If a patient has high-risk NMIBC, follow-up should be more intensive given risks of progression. Although urine cytology has historically been thought to be specific for bladder cancer, a recent review has demonstrated low specificity for low-grade tumors, with an increase in specificity for high-grade tumors.[9] This limits the usefulness for urine cytology to high-grade tumor follow-up. Patients with high-grade NMIBC will have cystoscopy and cytology every 3 months for the first 2 years, then every 6 months for 2 years, and then annually (**Table 2**).[8]

Table 1
Initial management of non–muscle-invasive bladder cancer based on risk level

Risk	Initial	Ongoing
Low risk	Single installation of intravesical chemotherapy	None
Intermediate risk	Installation of intravesical chemotherapy	Maintenance intravesical chemotherapy × 1 y
High Risk	Intravesical BGC	Intravesical BCG × 3 y

Data from Kamat AM, Hahn NM, Efstathiou JA, et al. Bladder cancer. Lancet 2016;388:2796–810.

Table 2
Surveillance of non–muscle-invasive bladder cancer

Risk	Cystoscopy	Cytology
Low risk	At 3 mo, 1 y, and then annually	Not recommended
Intermediate risk[a]	Cystoscopy at 3 mo, cystoscopy every 3–4 mo × 2 y, every 6 mo × 1 y, then annually	
High risk	At 3 mo, then every 3 mo × 2 y, every 6 mo × 2 y, then annually	At 3 mo, then every 3 mo × 2 y, every 6 mo × 2 y, then annually

[a] Intermediate-risk patients may follow surveillance of low-risk or high-risk patients or as above, depending on risk factors.

Data from Chang SS, Bochner BH, Chour R, et al. Treatment of non-metastatic muscle invasive bladder cancer: AUA/ASCO/ASTRO/SUO guideline. Linthicum (MD): American Urological Association; 2017.

Treatment of MIBC is surgical and surveillance is indicated to look for recurrent disease, new lesions in the upper urinary tract, and complications such as hydronephrosis. Surveillance of MIBC should include cross-sectional imaging of the abdomen and pelvis every 6 months for 3 years and then annually (**Table 3**). Laboratory work includes evaluation of renal function and electrolytes every 3 to 6 months for 3 years. Cytology is not recommended for surveillance, given that the bladder should have been surgically removed as part of the treatment plan.[8] After surgical treatment of bladder cancer, primary care physicians should monitor a patient's overall tolerance of this procedure. Patients may need assistance with continence, sexual health, and body image.

KIDNEY CANCER

Renal cancer is the sixth most common cancer in men in and the 10th most common cancer in women in the United States, with 5% of all new cancer diagnoses in men and 3% of all new cancer diagnoses in women being attributed to kidney cancer.[1] Kidney cancer is estimated to cause 3% of cancer deaths in men each year with men 1.5 times more likely to develop renal cancer than women. Developed countries have higher incidences of renal cancer than developing countries due to risk factors of smoking, obesity, and hypertension.[1]

Renal cell carcinoma (RCC) can arise from the renal parenchyma or the renal pelvis. By far the most common renal cancer is adenocarcinoma of the renal parenchyma, which accounts for more than 90% of all renal cancers.[11] RCCs are most commonly clear-cell type, then papillary, then chromophore tumors.[11]

Table 3
Surveillance of muscle-invasive disease

Laboratory	Radiology	Cytology/Cystoscopy
Renal function test every 3–6 mo × 3 y	Computed tomography/ MRI abdomen/pelvis every 3–6 mo	Not done

Data from Chang SS, Bochner BH, Chour R, et al. Treatment of non-metastatic muscle invasive bladder cancer: AUA/ASCO/ASTRO/SUO guideline. Linthicum (MD): American Urological Association; 2017.

On diagnosis of RCC, most patients will have disease confined to one kidney. If the disease is metastatic, the lungs, bone, and brain are the most common site of metastasis.[12]

Risk Factors and Screening

The most common risk factors for renal cancer include cigarette smoking, hypertension, and obesity. However, these may not be well understood as risk factors by the general public.[13]

Cigarette smoking has been found to increase the risk of renal cancer in both men and woman. Male smokers have a 50% increased risk of developing RCC, whereas female smokers have only a 20% increased risk of developing renal carcinoma compared with their nonsmoking counterparts.[12] It is believed that the increased risk comes from an element of chronic tissue hypoxia, rather than from the nicotine or tobacco itself. The risk of renal cancer increases with length of exposure and amount of pack years, whereas smoking cessation decreases risk.

Obesity and excess body weight have been estimated to account for 40% of RCCs in the United States. Risk of developing RCC is increased with increasing body mass index.[12]

Hypertension is also noted to be a risk factor. Elevated blood pressure causes chronic renal hypoxia, which leads to the increased risk. Appropriate control of blood pressure decreases risk of developing kidney cancer.[12]

Diabetes, dialysis, and lack of exercise have been postulated, but not conclusively demonstrated to be risk factors. Occupational exposure is not a proven risk at this time.[12]

Screening

There is currently no recommended screening for renal cancer, including in patients with elevated risk.

Clinical Presentation

It is rare that a physician will make a diagnosis of RCC based on a patient's presentation. The clinical presentation and workup are described as follows; however, it is far more likely that renal cancer diagnosis will be made during the workup of an incidental mass on imaging. Most frequently, the family doctor will be presented with an incidental kidney mass found on imaging and will need to perform workup and referral based on these results.[14]

Only 30% of renal cancer diagnoses are made based on clinical presentation of a symptomatic patient.[12] When patients present with symptoms, they are typically vague and nonspecific such as acute or chronic flank pain or hematuria.[12] Paraneoplastic symptoms, including hypertension, anemia, polycythemia, hypercalcemia or weight loss, are common presenting concerns for 10% to 20% of patients with metastatic disease.[15] Hypertension may be difficult to discern, as a paraneoplastic symptom opposed to a chronic condition. There are no pathognomonic findings for a localized renal mass on physical examination. Physical findings are usually indicative of metastatic or advanced disease, and include adenopathy, grade III varicocele, body habitus, and physical findings of chronic kidney disease.[12] There is no biomarker useful in diagnosing renal carcinoma, but the AUA recommends considering laboratory workup for evaluation of metastatic disease and to evaluate renal function.[12,15]

Imaging to evaluate for staging is based primarily on patient's symptoms at the time of evaluation. **Box 1** summarizes recommended laboratory workup and imaging. A chest radiograph (CXR) is done routinely to assist with staging, but further radiologic images are based on a patient's symptoms. At this time, the AUA does not

Box 1
Suggested routine workup of renal mass

Laboratory	CBC, CMP, UA
Imaging	CXR
Further imaging (based on symptoms)	
Pulmonary symptoms	Chest CT
Bone pain	Bone scan
Neurologic symptoms	Brain imaging (CT or MRI)

Abbreviations: CBC, complete blood count; CMP, comprehensive metabolic panel; CT, computed tomography; CXR, chest radiograph; UA, urinalysis.

Data from Campbell S, Uzzo R, Allaf M, et al. Renal mass and localized renal cancer: AUA guideline. Linthicum (MD): American Urological Association; 2017; and Rini B, McKiernan J, Chang S, et al. Kidney. In: Amin MB, editor. AJCC cancer staging manual. 8th edition. Chicago: Springer; 2017. p. 739–48.

recommend a PET scan for evaluation or staging of RCC, as the kidneys have a high background uptake.[15,16]

Radiologic Diagnosis of Renal Masses

Incidental renal masses are a common finding on imaging that most family physicians will need to evaluate during their time in practice. With the vast availability of advanced imaging, an incidental renal lesion can be identified on 13% to 27% of abdominal imaging studies.[17] Even though most incidental renal masses are benign, differentiating a benign incidental finding from a malignant mass is critical for proper management.

Incidental renal masses can be seen on ultrasound imaging, CT scan, or MRI. Renal masses are divided into cystic and solid types. Cystic masses are classified by the Bosniak classification, and solid masses are evaluated on size. Aside from simple renal cysts (classified as Bosniak I), all renal masses seen as an incidental finding, both cystic and solid, need to be fully evaluated with a dedicated renal CT with and without contrast or a dedicated MRI with and without gadolinium enhancement.[17,18] For both cystic and solid masses, a radiologic finding of enhancement of the lesion on the MRI or CT scan are concerning and must be considered malignant until proven otherwise.[17]

The Bosniak classification for cystic masses of the kidney was developed in 1986 and has undergone updates with improvements in imaging. The Bosniak classification system is used on renal cystic masses on CT or MRI studies to assess level of concern and further follow-up needed. The Bosniak scoring system is detailed in **Table 4**. Bosniak I and II are likely benign and require no follow-up assessment, unless the patient is to develop symptoms of hematuria or flank pain.[19] Bosniak IIF (F designation indicating needs further follow-up), III, and IV are more concerning and need further assessment.

For solid renal masses, imaging is nondiagnostic for determining a benign versus a malignant mass; however, the size of the lesion can also lend to level of concern. For solid renal masses that are less than 1 cm, nearly half (46%) are benign (**Table 5**). Similarly, 22% of lesions 1.0 to 2.9 cm are benign, whereas only 20% of lesions 3.0 to 3.9 cm are benign. Of the masses that are malignant, large size correlates with higher pathologic grade.[17]

Management of Renal Masses

Although Bosniak I and II cystic structures are benign and need no further follow-up, patients with Bosniak IIF, III, or IV lesions or a solid mass of any size should be referred

Table 4
Description of Bosniak classification

Bosniak Classification	Terminology	Description	Further Workup	Rate of Malignancy
I	Simple cyst	Benign simple cyst with thin wall, no septa, no calcification, no solid component, no enhancement.	No follow-up	Very rare
II	Mildly complex benign cyst	Benign minimally complicated cyst that may contain hairline septa. Smooth, hairline calcifications. No enhancement.	No follow-up	Very rare
IIF	Moderately complex cyst	Cyst wall: minimal regular thickening. Multiple, minimally smooth septa. Thick, nodular calcification. No enhancement.	CT W&WO or MRI W&WO at 3, 6, 12 mo, then annually × 5 y	5%–15%
III	Indeterminate complex cyst	Cyst wall: irregular thickening. Thick, irregular septa. Thick irregular calcification. Enhances.	CT W&WO or MRI W&WO at 3, 6, 12 mo, then annually × 5 y OR surgical resection	40%–60%
IV	Complex cystic mass	Cyst wall: irregular thickening. Irregular gross thickened septa. Thick, nodular and irregular septa. Enhancing tissue and cyst.	Surgical resection	>80%

Abbreviations: CT, computed tomography; W&WO, with and without.
Data from Refs.[14,20,21]

Table 5
Percentage of malignancy by lesion size

Size of Lesion, cm	Percent Benign	Percent Malignant	Percent High Grade	Percent Locally Invaded	Percent with Metastasis
<1.0	54	46			
1.0–2.9	22	78			
3.0–3.9	20	80	14 –26	12 –36	1 –8

Data from Gill I, Aron M, Gervais D, et al. Small renal mass. N Engl J Med 2010;326(7):624–34.

to urology for further evaluation and management. The interdisciplinary team involved in care of patients with RCC may also include a nephrologist, interventional radiologist, pathologist, medical oncologist, and genetic counselor.[15]

Treatment

For solid masses or Bosniak III/IV masses, the urologist will review the 4 treatment options with the patients, which are (1) radical nephrectomy, (2) partial nephrectomy, (3) thermal ablation, and (4) active surveillance. Each of the 4 treatment options has its own risks and benefits, and treatment will be dependent on the patient's risk factors and clinical status going into treatment.[15]

Surgery has remained the standard treatment at this time, due to uncertainties of assessing malignancy via imaging alone, as well as a limited ability for clinicians to identify benign or malignant lesions on active surveillance of masses by imaging.[18,20,21]

Radial nephrectomy is a procedure that involves removal of the entire kidney and can be performed laparoscopically. This approach is preferred when the tumor is complex or large. Radical nephrectomy is associated with a low risk of urologic complications following the procedure; however, it does have a higher risk of leaving the patient with a decrease in glomerular filtration rate.[15]

Partial nephrectomy involves removing a portion of the kidney, and has a lower risk of decrease in kidney function, but has a higher risk of urologic complications such as urine leak, and a higher risk of blood transfusion needed during surgery.[15] The value of lymph node sampling in RCC is small in tumors less than 4 cm, making a partial nephrectomy without lymph node sampling an acceptable treatment for small tumors.[22]

Thermal ablation is a relatively new procedure, but has shown to be a consideration for small solid masses in select patients.[14] Thermal ablation is currently not recommended by the AUA in cystic masses until further studies are completed.[15]

Renal mass biopsy is an option for assisting with management and determination of malignancy, but does have limitations. Renal mass biopsy is considered a safe procedure with low risks for complications, has good sensitivity and specificity, and a positive predictive value of 99.8%. However, biopsy also has a concerning negative predictive value with as many as 37% of lesions that were benign on biopsy found to be malignant after excision.[15]

Active surveillance can be considered in patients who cannot tolerate a surgical procedure or in patients with limited life expectancy.[14,15] Studies have demonstrated very good survival rates for small solid masses that are followed for up to 3 years with no growth. Generally, surveillance will include imaging with CT, MRI or ultrasound every 3 to 6 months to assess for changes in the mass. A renal biopsy may be considered during the period of active management. A yearly CXR is recommended to assess for metastasis. The AUA also describes "expectant management," which is less intense

Table 6
Staging of kidney cancer

Stage	T	N	M	5-y Survival, %
I	T1	N0	M0	81
II	T2	N0	M0	74
III	T1 or T2	N1	M0	53
	T3	N0 or N1	M0	
IV	T4	Any N	M0	8
	Any T	Any N	M1	

Data from Rini B, McKiernan J, Chang S, et al. Kidney. In: Amin MB, editor. AJCC cancer staging manual. 8th edition. Chicago: Springer; 2017. p. 739–48; and American Cancer Society. Survival rates for kidney cancer by stage. Available at: https://www.cancer.org/cancer/kidney-cancer/detection-diagnosis-staging/survival-rates.html. Accessed July 1, 2018.

radiologic follow-up, and generally used for patients who will not be able to undergo treatment.[15]

Although guidelines for surveillance of renal masses is limited at this time, a recent study indicates that overtreatment of benign lesions often occurs. Resection of Bosniak III lesions is considered standard of care; however, as many as 50% of these lesions are found to be benign when removed.[20]

Surgical treatments are generally considered curative for localized disease, although chemotherapy, immunotherapy, or targeted therapy may be considered in recurrent or metastatic disease (**Table 6**).

SUMMARY

Bladder and renal cancer are common forms of cancer in the United States. Although no screening is recommended for either at this time, there are modifiable risk factors that primary care physicians should discuss with patients. Primary care providers should be familiar with the workup of hematuria and incidental renal masses, and be prepared to support patients through treatment.

REFERENCES

1. Siegel R, Miller K, Jemal A. Cancer statistics, 2018. CA Cancer J Clin 2018;68: 7–30.
2. Bochner B, Hansel D, Efstathiou J, et al. Urinary bladder. AJCC cancer staging manual. 8th edition 2017. p. 757–65.
3. Kamat AM, Hahn NM, Efstathiou JA, et al. Bladder cancer. Lancet 2016;388: 2796–810.
4. Chang SS, Boorjian SA, Chou R, et al. Diagnosis and treatment of non-muscle invasive bladder cancer: AUA/SUO Guideline. J Urol 2016;196(4):1021–9.
5. Burger M, Catto J, Dalbagni G. Epidemiology and risk factors of urothelial bladder cancer. Eur Urol 2013;16:234–41.
6. Antoni S, Ferlay J, Soerjomataram I, et al. Bladder cancer incidence and mortality: a global overview and recent trends. Eur Urol 2017;71:96–108.
7. Chou R, Dana T. Screening adults for bladder cancer: a review of the evidence for the U.S. preventive services task force. Ann Intern Med 2010;153(7):461–8.
8. Chang SS, Bochner BH, Chour R, et al. Treatment of non-metastatic muscle invasive bladder cancer: AUA/ASCO/ASTRO/SUO guideline. American Urological Association (AUA)/American Society of Clinical Oncology (ASCO)/American

Society for Radiation Oncology (ASTRO)/Society of Urologic Oncology (SUO). J Urol 2017;198(3):552–9.
9. Bellmunt J, Orsola A, Leow JJ, et al. Bladder cancer: EMSO practice guidelines for diagnosis, treatment and follow up. Ann Oncol 2014;(Supplement 3):iii40–8.
10. Kassouf W, Traboulsi S, Schmitz-Drager B, et al. Follow-up in non-muscle-invasive bladder cancer-International Bladder Cancer Network recommendations. Urol Oncol 2016;34:460–8.
11. Chow W, Dong L, Devesa S. Epidemiology and risk factors for kidney cancer. Nat Rev Urol 2010;7(5):245–57.
12. Capitanio U, Montorsi F. Renal cancer. Lancet 2016;387(10021):894–906.
13. Parker A, Arnold M, Diehl N, et al. Evaluation and awareness of risk factors for kidney cancer among patients presenting to a urology clinic. Scand J Urol 2014;48:239–44.
14. Babian K, Delacroix S, Wood C, et al. Kidney cancer. Brenner's and Rector's the kidney. Philadelphia, PA: Elsevier; 2016.
15. Campbell S, Uzzo R, Allaf M, et al. Renal mass and localized renal cancer: AUA guideline. J Urol 2017;198(3):520–9.
16. Rini B, McKiernan J, Chang S, et al. Kidney. AJCC cancer staging manual. 8th edition 2017. p. 739–48.
17. Gill I, Aron M, Gervais D, et al. Small renal mass. N Engl J Med 2010;326(7): 624–34.
18. Herts B, Silverman S, Hindman N, et al. Management of the incidental renal mass on CT: a white paper of the ACR incidental findings committee. J Am Coll Radiol 2018;15:264–73.
19. Simms R, Ong A. How simple are 'simple renal cysts'? Nephrol Dial Transplant 2014;29:iv106–12.
20. Schoots I, Zaccai K, Hunink M, et al. Bosniak classification for complex renal cysts revaluated: a systemic review. J Urol 2017;198:12–21.
21. Lam C, Kapoor A. The true malignancy risk of Bosniak III cystic renal lesions: active surveillance or surgical resection? Can Urol Assoc J 2018;12(6):E276–80.
22. Mirza K, Taxy J, Antic T. Radical nephrectomy for renal cell carcinoma. Am J Clin Pathol 2016;145:837–42.

Printed and bound by CPI Group (UK) Ltd, Croydon, CR0 4YY
03/10/2024
01040403-0006